THE UNRAVELLING

Clem Martini & Olivier Martini

How our caregiving safety net came
unstrung and we were left grasping at
threads, struggling to plait a new one

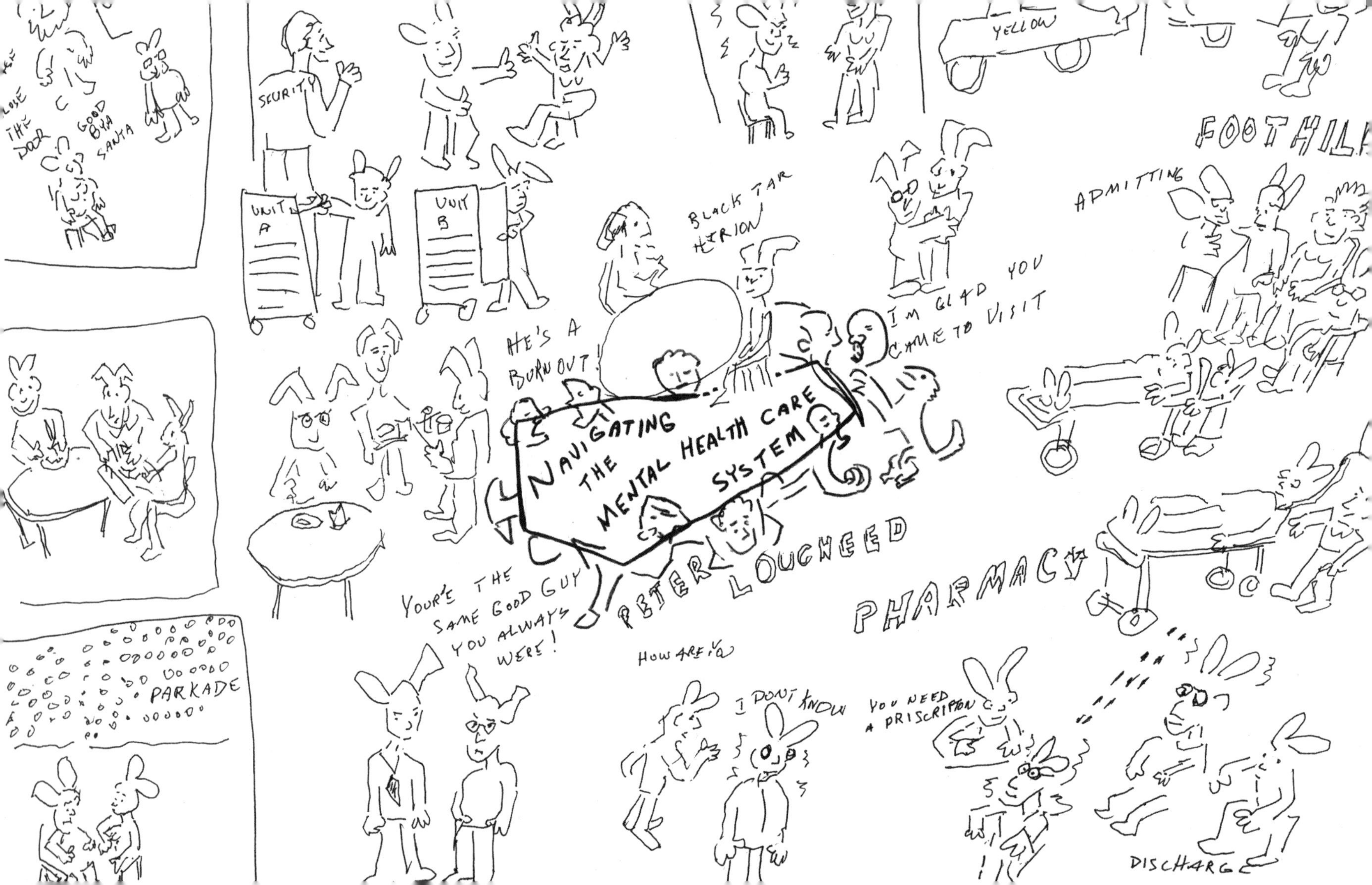
NAVIGATING THE MENTAL HEALTH CARE SYSTEM
PETER LOUGHEED
FOOTHILL
ADMITTING
PHARMACY
PARKADE
DISCHARGE
YELLOW
SECURITY
UNIT A
UNIT B
BLACK TAR HERION
HE'S A BURNOUT!
I'M GLAD YOU CAME TO VISIT
YOU'RE THE SAME GOOD GUY YOU ALWAYS WERE!
HOW ARE YOU
I DON'T KNOW
YOU NEED A PRISCRIPTION
GOOD BYA SANTA

"If I had a world of my own, everything would be nonsense. Nothing would be what it is, because everything would be what it isn't. And contrary wise, what is, it wouldn't be. And what it wouldn't be, it would. You see?"

LEWIS CARROLL

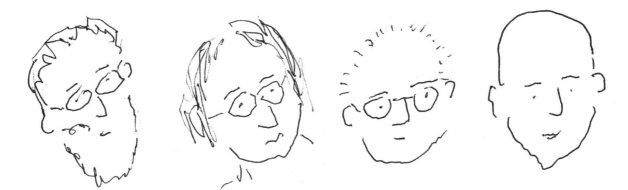

To deal with mental illnesses and dementia is to enter a mirror world, where words can often mean their opposite. Truth and lies can be exchanged, one for the other, and perhaps the most dangerous lies are the ones we tell ourselves.

Introduction

The Unravelling is the story of Liv and his family. Liv has schizophrenia. His mother, his caregiver of many years, is sinking into the abyss of dementia. His brothers, who provide ongoing support, pick up the pieces whenever the health care system fails. Who or what is unravelling in this story? Liv? His mother? His brothers? The system?

Caregiving can be complicated. In some cases the line between caregiver and recipient can be blurry. For years Liv's mother cared for him, and in return Liv provided emotional support, companionship, and physical help to her. What happens when the delicate balance is interrupted by the onset of ill health, old age, dementia, and the once reliable caregiver becomes care recipient? Other family members intensify their engagement, now caring for a brother with schizophrenia as well as a mother with several physical health issues and escalating dementia. Clem, Liv's brother and the narrator of this story, seems to sail through the murky waters of schizophrenia and dementia care with much poise. He is an experienced caregiver and knows how to navigate the system, but his endurance is tested times and again. Dementia, as Clem notes, "isn't a decline: it's a plummet from a precipice. And as you fall you strike against the rocky cliff face, each strike removing another portion of who you were." For Liv, the pain of losing his mother — his main support — to dementia, is compounded by the feeling that he has failed to take care of her.

With most of us, if not all, expected to be caregivers or care recipients at one time or another, and with the current state of health care throughout the country, the picture is bleak. This book is a testimony to the trials and tribulations of one family, whose patience and good will are exhausted by an unfriendly, often hostile health care system; it is also a manifesto against the priorities that create the many shortcomings of health and social services.

This very personal and intimate book is extraordinary in its description of ordinary situations. Accompanied by Liv's moving drawings, which are at once filled with compassion, confusion, fear, and at times humour, it is a must read for us all.

Ella Amir, Executive Director, AMI-Québec Action on Mental Ilness

Ella Amir has been working with families affected by mental illness since 1990 in her capacity as the Executive Director of the Montreal-based AMI-Quebec Action on Mental Illness. Ella was the chair of the former Family Caregivers Advisory Committee at the Mental Health Commission of Canada and is now a member of its Advisory Committee.

It's early and dark when the phone rings.

I haven't had breakfast yet and am just set up at the dining room table, papers strewn in front of me, picking at my computer keyboard and nursing a cup of warm tea. I lift the receiver, cradle it to my ear, and am surprised to hear my brother's psychiatrist on the other end. Dr. Baxter apologizes for calling early, tells me she has phoned Olivier's, and has been unable to reach him. Where is he?

His blood work has returned from the lab, she tells me, and there's a problem. The tests indicate his white blood cells have been seriously compromised. She mentions the possible condition he is suffering from — it's long and scary-sounding: agranulocytosis. It's essential that he get to emergency at once, she says.

I consider where he might be. Olivier is an early riser, and each morning he promptly flies out the door. Typically, his day is crammed full of visits to support groups, social agencies, and art clinics. I recall he had mentioned that he would be working on a sculpture in his art class at Self Help, a community mental health support centre.

I say I'll try to get hold of him there. She tells me she'll call the Foothills Hospital to prepare a placement for him.

The coordinator at Self Help says Olivier has just arrived so I ask her to bring him to the phone. When he picks up, I fill him in on the situation and tell him that I'll drive down and get him. The coordinator, who has overheard the conversation, interrupts to say she'll call a taxi to save time.

Liv and I meet at the hospital twenty minutes later. I steel myself to accompany him through emergency intake, which I tend to view as something like hell with all the good bits left out. There are the endless lineups: first you line up to receive an identification number and state your condition, then you line up again to see someone who will establish if the condition is serious, then you wait for someone to arrive who will actually examine you, and so on. There are the sad, angry, tortured souls haunting the waiting room, the feverish and the drunk, the bleeding and the nauseous. There are the chairs, designed to punish, and over everything hangs the smell of vomit blended with the sharp, piney odour of disinfectant.

So, now we wait.

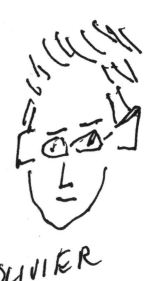

OLIVIER

An hour and a half later we're transferred into the examination area and a doctor arrives. He confirms what Liv's psychiatrist suspected: Olivier's white blood cell count has plummeted. The doctor is young and self-assured and not particularly adept at communicating. I ask a few questions. No, he doesn't know why this condition has suddenly appeared. No, he doesn't know what can be done. No, there are no beds available. It will be several hours before Liv can expect a placement, and I reflect that emergency, where every form of virus, germ, or bacteria collects, is the worst possible environment for someone with a compromised immune system.

Liv is conducted down a narrow corridor, provided with a temporary cot, and handed a sandwich wrapped in plastic and a juice pack — dinner. I ask him if he's okay. He says he is and I tell him I'll return in the morning — hopefully by then a bed will have been secured, and someone will be able to sort this all out.

When I get home I phone my mother to let her know that Olivier will likely spend the next few nights at the hospital, then I text my oldest brother, Nic, to let him know what's happened. He says he'll pay a visit to Olivier after work the next day. I sit down at my computer and Google *agranulocytosis.* Wikipedia offers this definition: "*People with this condition are at very high risk of serious infections due to their suppressed immune system.*" Any number of small problems can quickly advance and become dangerous.

It "*may clinically present with sudden fever, rigors, and sore throat. Infection of any organ may be rapidly progressive (e.g. pneumonia, urinary tract infection). Septicemia may also progress rapidly.*"

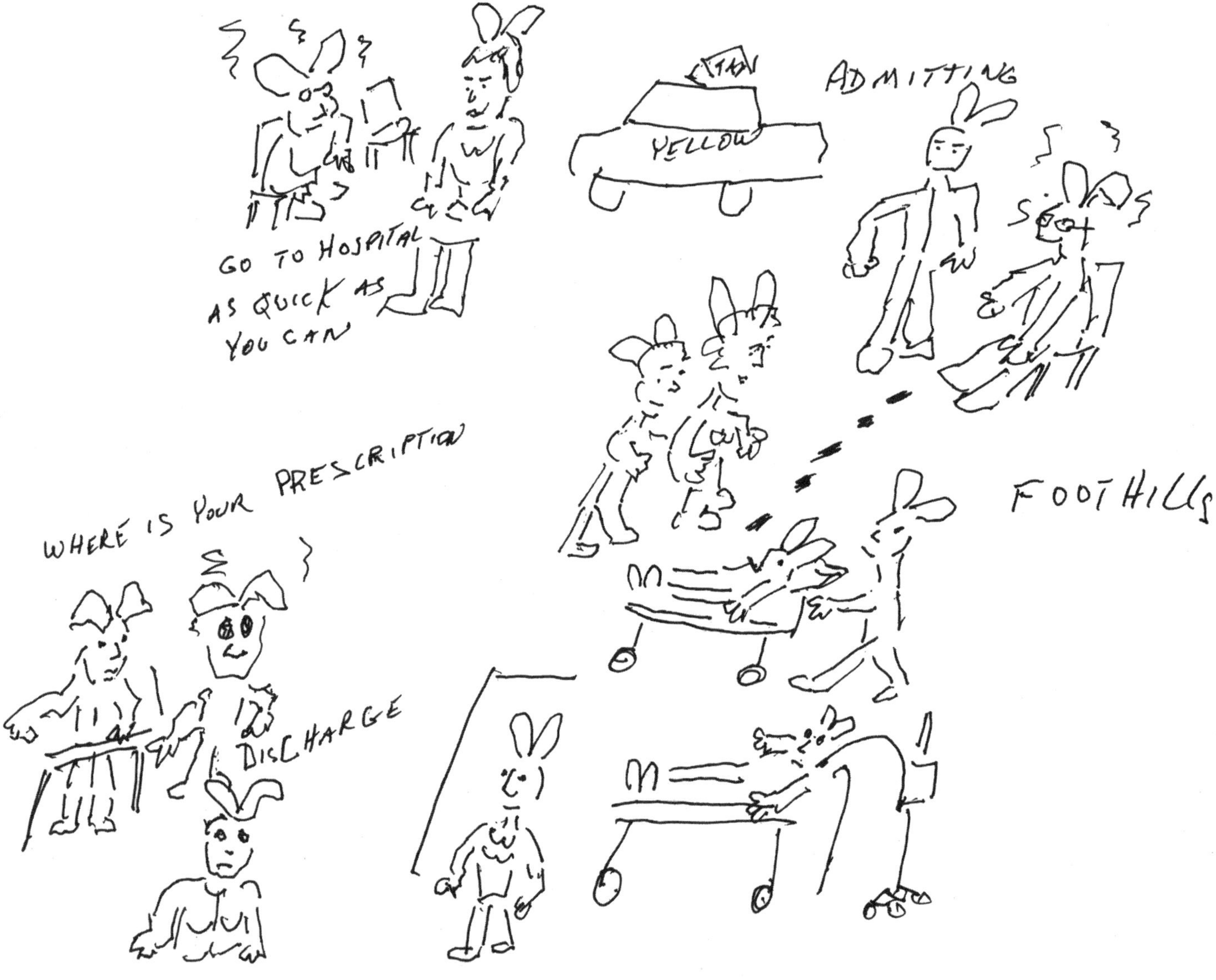
GO TO HOSPITAL
AS QUICK AS
YOU CAN
TAXI
YELLOW
ADMITTING
FOOTHILLS
WHERE IS YOUR PRESCRIPTION
DISCHARGE

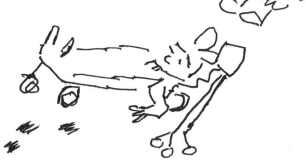

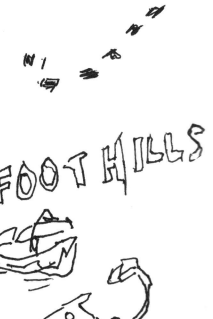

FOOT HILLS

When I get home I tell my wife, Cheryl, what's happened. She's sympathetic, but assures me there's nothing to be done till Liv has received a full examination. And she's right, but when I go to bed I can't sleep. I keep returning to Liv's blood problems. I'd noticed that something was wrong with Liv over a month ago. He'd seemed unusually tired and confused. When I brought breakfast over for Liv and Mom, he would eat it, finish, and flake out on the couch.

I'd interpreted this as another side effect of his meds, and had asked him to consult with his doctor. He assured me that he'd do so, but who knows if he did? Or maybe he did, and the doctor didn't follow up. In any case, I should have stayed on it. Obviously, I'd dropped the ball.

I rise early, eat, and return to the hospital. Liv has at last been transferred from emergency to internal medicine, the hematology unit, which is troubling. I'd hoped that he would be treated in the psychiatric unit where they would have a better understanding not only of his medical history but also the complications associated with mental illness. During his thirty-plus-years-long experience with schizophrenia, Liv has developed a relationship with staff at most of the psychiatric facilities in the city. When I get to Liv's room, I'm introduced to the attending medical specialist: a youngish man accompanied by an even younger someone else in training. It's clear to me from our first few minutes of conversation that they don't know how to deal with Olivier or me.

They understand both from Olivier's chart and from his confused responses that he has a mental illness. You can see from the way they more or less ignore Olivier that they don't view him as entirely competent, so they don't run everything by him, but they're reticent to share things with me as they don't view me as having any genuine standing in the situation either. As a consequence, they simply chat amongst themselves and never really consult either of us.

Apparently, the length of my brother's list of prescription medication makes things complicated. The doctors don't really know which drug, or combination of drugs, is responsible for his condition, but from what I've read the primary suspect seems to be clozapine. There's a sufficiently high incidence of agranulocytosis among people prescribed the drug that they are required to take ongoing monthly blood tests. I voice my concern about what the next steps might involve, because Olivier has had a long and difficult experience with other antipsychotics – they either haven't worked or have had severe side effects. If clozapine is no longer an option, what will he do?

The doctors caution me not to jump to conclusions. The way they'll probably proceed will be to remove one drug at a time from Liv's system, observe the results, and go from there. This sounds complicated, and I prepare for the possibility that my brother will be in the hospital a long while.

I AM GOING TO THE PHARMACY

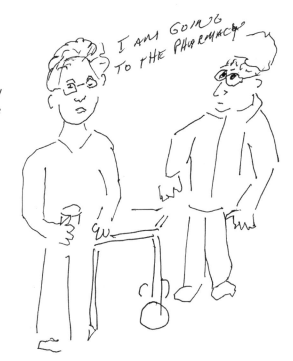

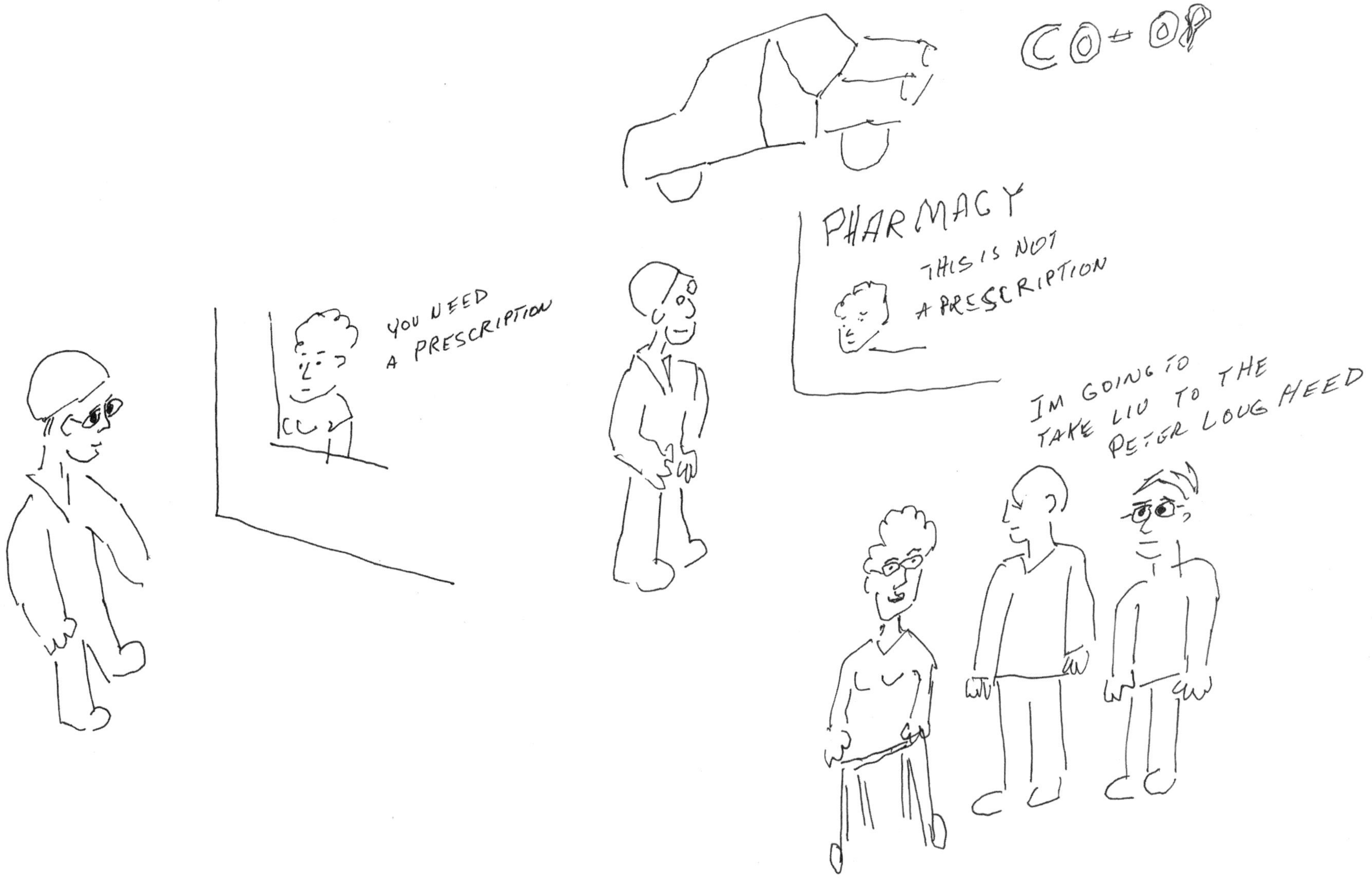
CO-OP
PHARMACY
THIS IS NOT A PRESCRIPTION
YOU NEED A PRESCRIPTION
IM GOING TO TAKE LIU TO THE PETER LOUGHEED

Three days later I receive another early morning call. Can I come and get him, Liv asks. He's been released.

I'm caught completely off guard. When I'd visited Liv the previous night, I hadn't received any indication that the doctors had even determined which drug was the culprit. He tells me that he'll be waiting downstairs. I fire a quick email to Dr. Baxter asking if she knows what's going on, then throw on a jacket.

I find him at the main entrance to the Foothills Hospital, his jacket on, his suitcase packed, seated among the old, ill men and women who sprawl in their hospital gowns, IVs attached to their arms. He stands, detaches himself from the throng, slides into the passenger side, and shuts the door.

"Is everything all right?" I ask as he buckles himself in.

"I guess so," he says.

That doesn't sound reassuring. "What did the doctors say?"

"That my blood levels were good and then they kicked me out."

"How come they didn't tell you that you'd be released last night?" I ask. "Why wasn't there more warning?"

"I don't know," he says.

I can't believe that given the degree of risk his previous condition held, there hasn't been some kind of advice or follow-up. "Is there anything you should be doing to prevent this from happening again?" I ask.

"They didn't tell me," he replies.

"And you didn't receive any written information?" I ask.

"Nope, they said they'd forward something on to my doctor."

I pull out of the loading bay and glance over at Liv. He still sounds tired to me, but maybe that's not surprising. I only have to visit a hospital for an hour to feel exhausted. He remains quiet during the drive home. I ask if he's sure he's okay. He nods.

I park the car and as he gets out I tell him I'll call later. When I arrive home I receive an email from his psychiatrist.

"Ok — I am blown away that the Foothills has discharged Olivier without talking to me!! I guess they at least had the courtesy of faxing me the discharge summary."

Luckily, she has an appointment to see Olivier the following morning, so she will be able to follow up with him then.

Later that night my mother calls, concerned about Olivier. He still doesn't seem himself, she says, but she seems somewhat reassured when I tell her that he is scheduled to meet with Dr. Baxter the next morning.

But the next morning I receive another email from Dr. Baxter.

"He missed his appointment," she says, "so I called him. He was clearly not himself. Unfortunately, I am out of the country for the next 2.5 weeks starting tomorrow evening, so the timing is terrible. I will check my email daily though so we can try to manage this and I will see him on my first day back —

Mon Dec 9 at 5pm. If you were able to accompany Olivier to that appointment, that would be helpful. The Sheldon Chumir contacted me yesterday and stated they would be unwilling to help with any follow-up as Olivier lives in the NW *(they've changed the rules about how the clinics work) and that if any additional mental health supports are required, he will need to attend the* NW *clinic and there is a wait-list. So, we're on our own."*

I don't much like any of the content of that email, and particularly don't like the portion where she says "we're on our own." She concludes . . .

"Worst-case scenario, if Olivier is continuing to decline, please just take him to the ER and ask for a psychiatric hospital admission."

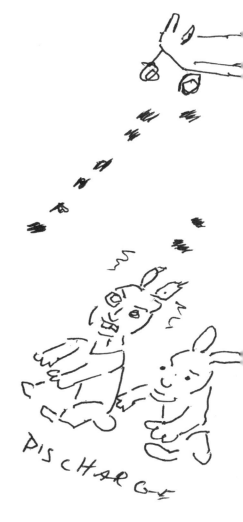

PISCHARGE

Fantastic. Olivier will be off at his various appointments throughout the day, but I make a mental note to call him later in the evening to find out what's happening.

I've just finished dinner when my mother calls. "Something is definitely wrong with Olivier."

"Something?" I ask. "What?"

"I don't know," she says, "but he is acting so strange. He won't do anything."

"What do you mean, 'do'?" I ask, puzzled. I hear her call his name, and then after a pause she calls him again. Then she comes back on the line.

"Here," she says, "you speak to him." I hear the rustle of the phone being passed from one hand to another.

"Hello?" I say.

There's a pause and then Olivier says, "Hello?"

"What's going on?" No answer. "Hello?" I say again.

Another long pause, then he says, "Hello?"

"Liv?" I say.

Silence.

"Give the phone to Mom," I tell him.

Nothing.

"Give the phone to Mom, Liv."

When there's still no response I shout, "Mom, take the phone!"

"You see," she says, once she's back on the line.

"I'm coming over," I tell her, and hang up.

I DONT KNOW THE RIGHT ANSWER

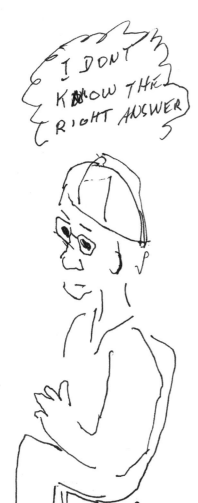

"There," my mother says, ushering me into the living room and gesturing at my brother with her cane, "you see."

Normally Olivier would turn to greet me, but he's seated on a chair, staring straight ahead.

"I can't make any sense of it," she tells me.

I approach him. "Hi Liv, what's the matter?"

He slowly turns. He seems aware of me, at least I think he is aware of me, but he doesn't answer.

"Liv?" I unzip my jacket, feeling suddenly hot. "Are you all right?"

His face is fixed in an odd expression, as though he detects my presence, but doesn't recognize me. And it's not just me he doesn't recognize: it's like he's viewing the entire world for the first time and can't sort it out. His eyes are stretched open extra wide. He blinks and glances about as though trying to process new information. I've seen Liv experiencing a mental crisis a number of times, but this is something totally new.

"Can you hear me?" I ask. He doesn't respond. "Liv, can you hear me?"

"Yes," he answers without conviction after a long moment.

I send a text to Dr. Baxter to let her know that Liv is in serious trouble, then tell Olivier what she said in her last email. I ask him if he understands. He just considers me with that same absent expression. I tell him we're going to the hospital. He blinks. I haven't a clue how to proceed.

"Liv?"

Nothing.

"Liv?" I ask. "Can you follow me?"

He appears uncertain, then says, "Yes," and stands.

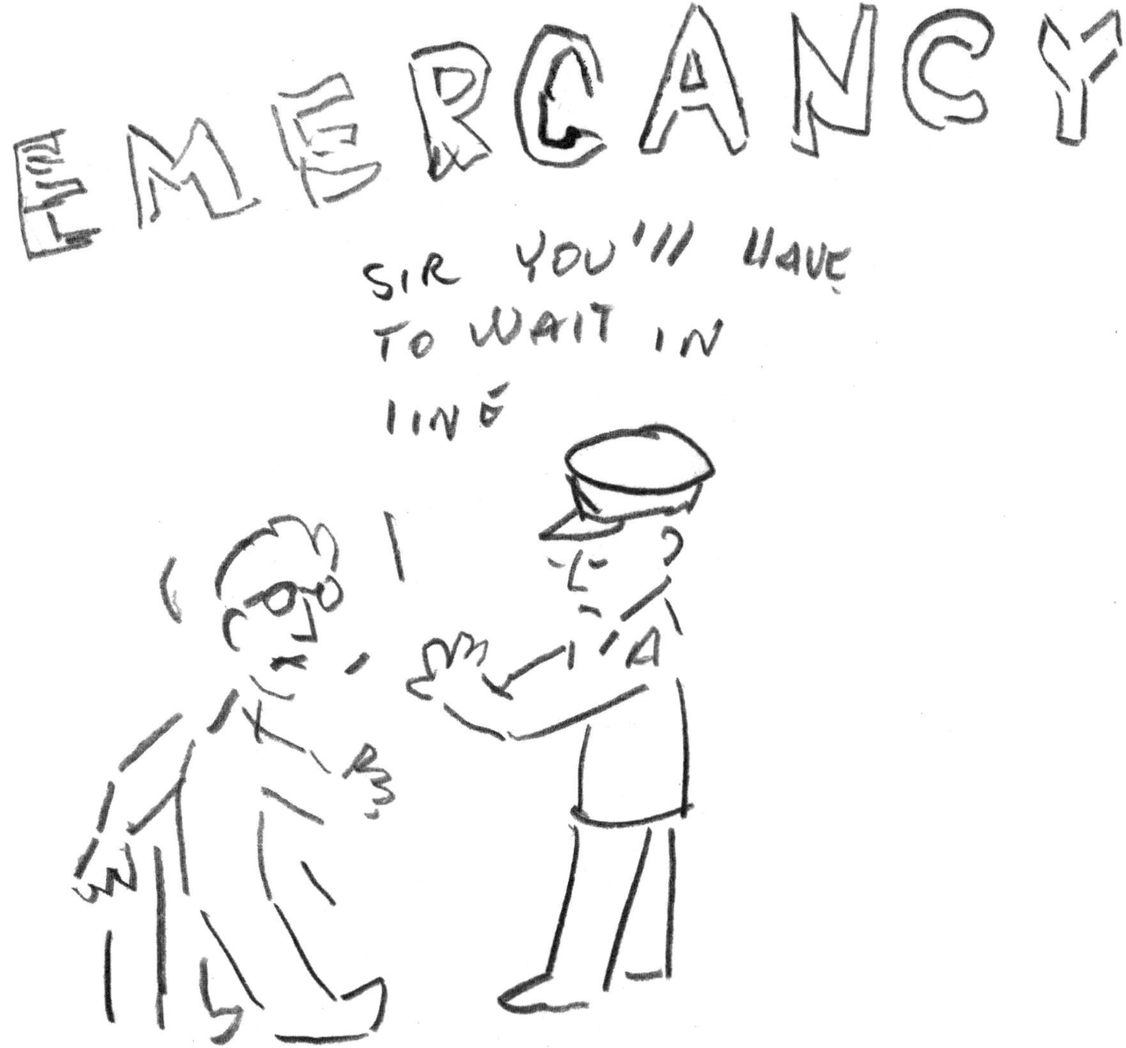
EMERGANCY
SIR YOU'LL HAVE TO WAIT IN LINE

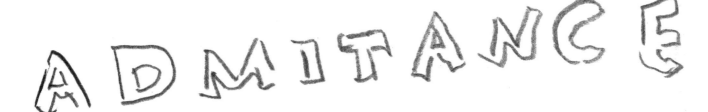

ADMITANCE

We arrive at the Lougheed Hospital, a big, grey, boxy institution, the kind of building that governments favour for hospitals and prisons. The parking lot is tiny and crowded. I wedge my car into the half space left to me after an SUV consumes a space-and-a-half, then slither out on the driver's side and lock the door. Together, Liv and I make our way toward the hospital.

Emergency intake again! Over the years this is where we have inevitably been directed whenever Liv has experienced a psychotic episode, but short of catapulting him through a fifth-storey window, I can't imagine a worse way for an individual experiencing psychiatric difficulties to enter a hospital system.

I coax him to follow me with words and hand signals but can't confirm how much gets through; nevertheless he trails after me, shuffling unsteadily.

At the emergency intake I try to explain the nature of the emergency to the person on duty. She brushes me off and tells me she wishes to speak to Olivier.

"Okay," I think, stepping back, "good luck."

Liv is, of course, unable to answer the most basic questions. A few minutes later, frustrated, she waves me back. I quickly sketch in the circumstances that led to my bringing him in, tell her that his psychiatrist has called ahead. Liv is provided a hospital identification bracelet, and we're told to sit.

We wait in the designated area, and because emergency is designed to prioritize cases according to how close you are to dying, and because no one has ever actually died as a result of a psychosis — at least while on the premises — we wait a considerable time. Four hours later we're escorted to an inner area, where we wait some more until someone again attempts to extract information, first from Liv and again, when that fails, from me. We linger in this new area for a little over an hour. An intern arrives to perform an intake interview with Olivier, reading from a lengthy checklist of formulaic mental health questions. I'm pretty sure that Olivier can't comprehend a single one of them. Frequently he doesn't reply, and the intern then repeats the question. Sometimes Olivier will offer, randomly, I believe, a quiet yes or no. One of the questions is whether he is contemplating self-harm.

The intern doesn't receive a response, and so asks again. Liv hesitantly answers yes.

And maybe he is. Or maybe he simply understands that a question of some kind has been posed and hopes this is the correct answer. In any case, we are now guided to a secure ward. This is all very discouraging. The way the hospital is handling my brother's crisis, and the nature of Olivier's illness itself. I've witnessed Olivier in various states of mental distress over the years, but never anything as severe. It's as though he has slipped through a crack into another dimension, and is only able to communicate through the thinnest fracture.

We pass our time in silence. Our new waiting area looks remarkably like a military bunker: compact, dimly lit, the walls unadorned apart from scuffs and scratches indicating a history of past conflict. The furnishings consist of a padded cot and a plastic chair. The door is sturdy and can be locked from outside. Luckily at this point it's been left open, otherwise the room would feel unbearably claustrophobic. In the room adjacent to ours, another client rages at his attendants and mutters angrily about killing people. I don't know what effect he has on my brother, but he terrifies me.

We wait. The traditional plastic-wrapped sandwiches are dropped off, accompanied by two juice boxes. Another man enters our room, this time a psychiatrist. He too directs questions at Olivier, which of course my brother still cannot answer, so I try to provide a quick rundown of Liv's last few weeks. I point out that this episode is quite different to previous relapses. The psychiatrist takes notes but doesn't waste much time soliciting additional information from me, which just confirms my every experience with the health care system as a relative of a person with a mental illness. I am present, but I am never *really* present. I am like the spectral Patrick Swayze character in the film *Ghost* — I can observe what's going on, but can't actually be seen or heard.

The psychiatrist finally looks at me and says they will try to find a bed for Olivier, but there are presently no openings. Does he know when a bed is likely to become available? He doesn't, he says, and leaves.

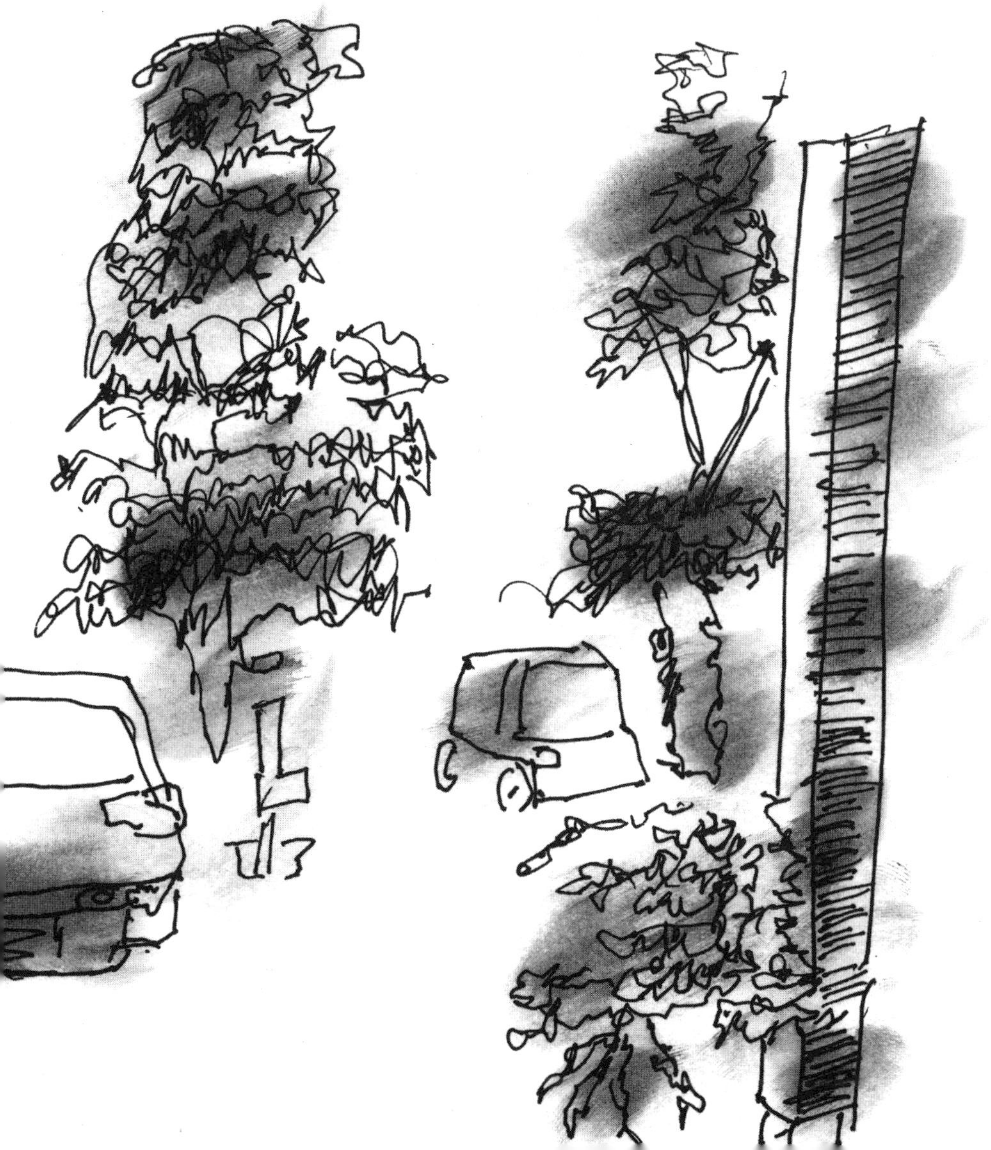

Time drags. The police arrive and take the angry man in the adjacent room away. I reflect on how strange the intake procedure must be for people suffering a psychiatric crisis. The environment, so uniformly grim and isolating, seems designed to promote depression and anxiety, rather than relieve it.

We wait. Olivier sleeps.

Finally, at 4:00 a.m., a bed is ready. I accompany Liv to the psychiatric unit. There, he's relieved of his belt, his wallet, his keys, his watch, and his comb. These personal articles are placed in a large manila envelope, his name written on the front with a black Sharpie.

I say good night to Olivier. He doesn't reply. The last sight I have of my brother as I exit the ward is of him seated on his bed, staring blankly ahead. I walk out to the parking lot, retrieve my car, and drive home in the dark.

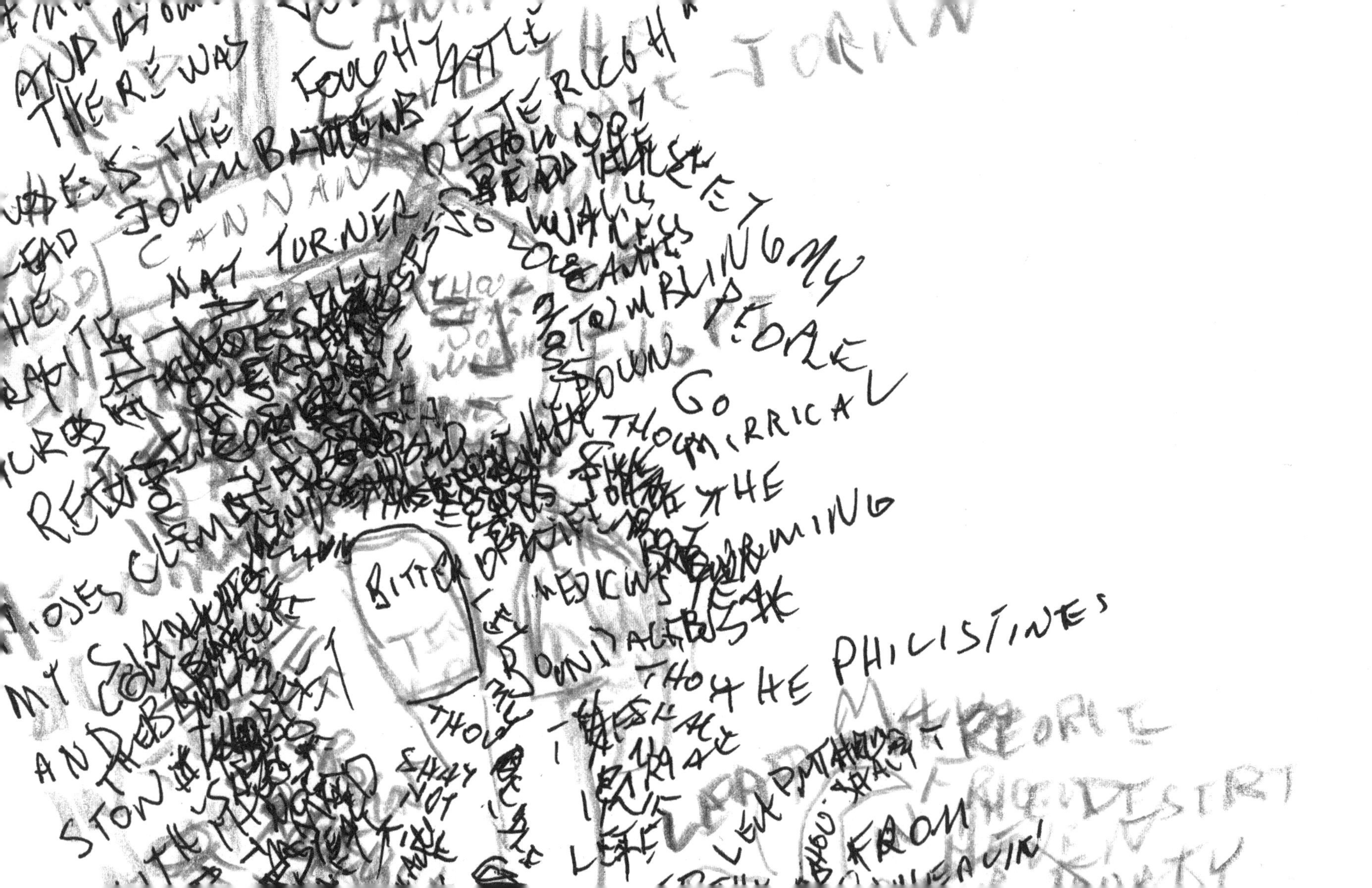

THERE WAS

JOHN BROWN FOUGHT BATTLE OF JERICOH JORDN

CANNAN

NAT TURNER

TUMBLING MY PEOPLE

GO THOU MIRRICAL

DOWN

THE BURNING

BITTER MEDICINE ROUND ABOUT

THEY THE PHILISTINES

MOSES CLEMENT

MY SLAVE AND COMPANY

STONE

PEOPLE FROM

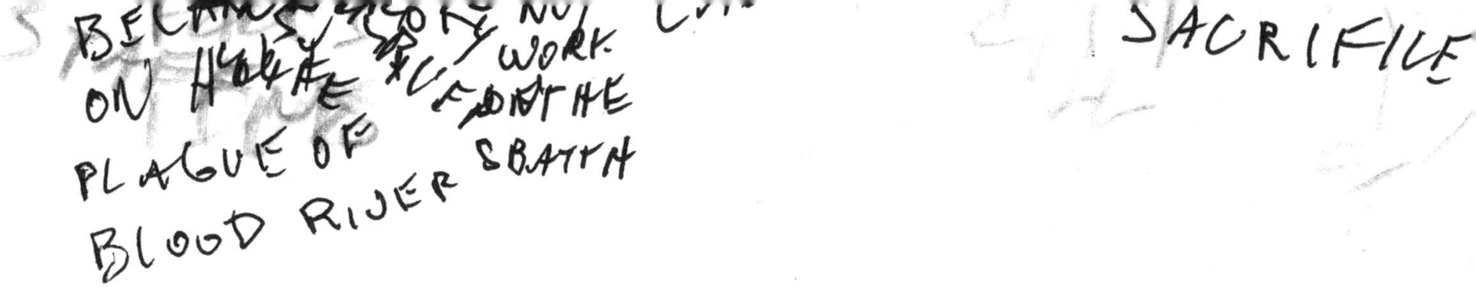
PLAGUE OF
BLOOD RIVER
SACRIFICE

Liv first showed signs of schizophrenia when he was twenty-six, only a few years after my younger brother, Ben, had been diagnosed with schizophrenia and then killed himself.

I was enrolled in Montreal's National Theatre School at the time, and my then-girlfriend (later to become my wife), Cheryl, called from Calgary to tell me that Liv was behaving oddly. The behaviours she described seemed to so exactly parallel Ben's earlier symptoms that I was stunned.

When I phoned to ask him what was going on he confessed that he had been feeling peculiar for months. He thought he was being followed by mysterious figures, was convinced he was receiving messages through the television. Sometimes he heard whispers that he was worthless and should just give up. I urged him to see a psychiatrist, but he told me he was too afraid. The doctors and hospitals all held places of prominence in his paranoid visions.

We agreed to stay in touch and monitor the situation, but after several long, anxious months the illness developed strength and power, and over the Christmas break Liv made an attempt on his life. This resulted in us driving in the middle of the night to the Holy Cross Hospital, where he checked into the psychiatric ward. December 23, 1980.

Ben's death had been terrible on so many different levels. Terrible because of how young he had been when it happened – only nineteen. Terrible because of its suddenness, because it was needless, because it was irrevocable. Then, Liv's diagnosis, following only a few years after, shook the whole family up badly. We wondered how we could move ahead not knowing if the disease could be cured or whether it would end in disaster, not knowing how to help, worried that we'd make a misstep. It was an enormous, complicated puzzle.

Thirty-six years later, my family is still trying to solve that puzzle.

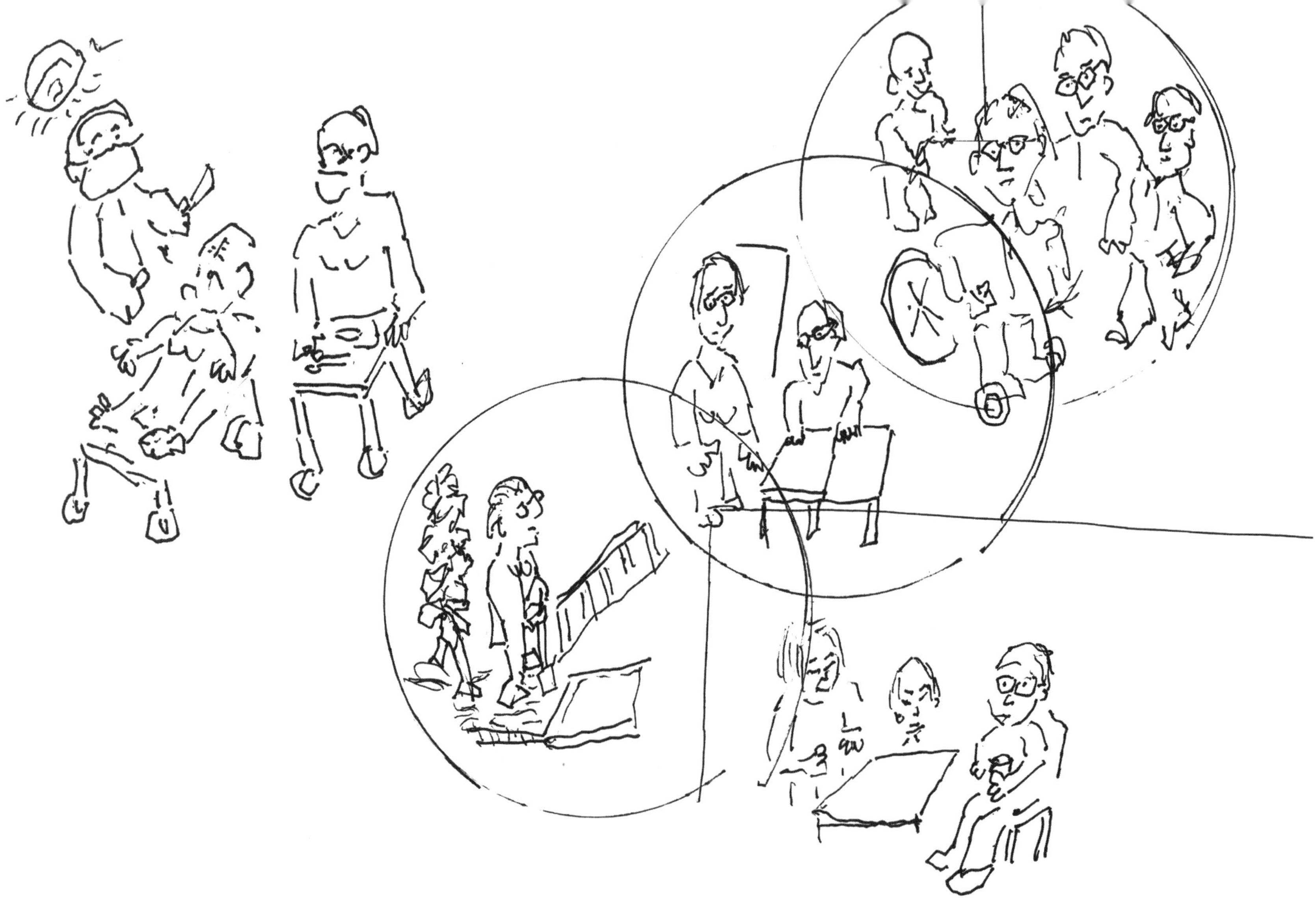

As soon as I get home, I text my oldest brother, Nic, updating him on Liv's situation and providing him with the hospital room number, then I phone my mother, knowing she will be worried. She and Olivier have lived together ever since his initial diagnosis thirty-six years ago. She's eighty-nine now, however, and in recent years their living situation has become more complex, as she has developed serious mobility issues. When she picks up, I give her a quick update, then say I'll drop by with breakfast after I've had a bit of sleep, and ask what time works best. She prides herself on being an early riser and answers that no matter when I arrive, she'll be up.

But at 7:00 a.m. when I let myself in, the apartment is dark. At first I think that she must still be in bed. Then I see a little light spilling from the open washroom door.

"Mom?" I call, to warn her that I've entered the apartment. It's a challenge to determine how loud to pitch my voice. Her hearing is poor, even with her hearing aids in, and she frequently doesn't install them until after she's had her first coffee. If I'm too quiet, she won't hear; if I'm too loud, she'll startle and maybe take a fall.

"Mom?" I call a bit louder. Nothing.

I close the door to the hallway and move toward the bathroom, where I find my mother staring at herself in the mirror. She's naked, so I step back.

"Hello?" I call to warn her, and when she doesn't respond, I say even louder, "Mom, are you okay?"

"No," she answers.

I step into the room. She is leaning forward, her arthritic hands gripping the lip of the sink, studying her reflection.

"Something's wrong," she replies in a voice so thick with either fear or pain, that at first I think she must be suffering a seizure or a stroke.

"What is? Mom?"

"I don't know," she says, still staring.

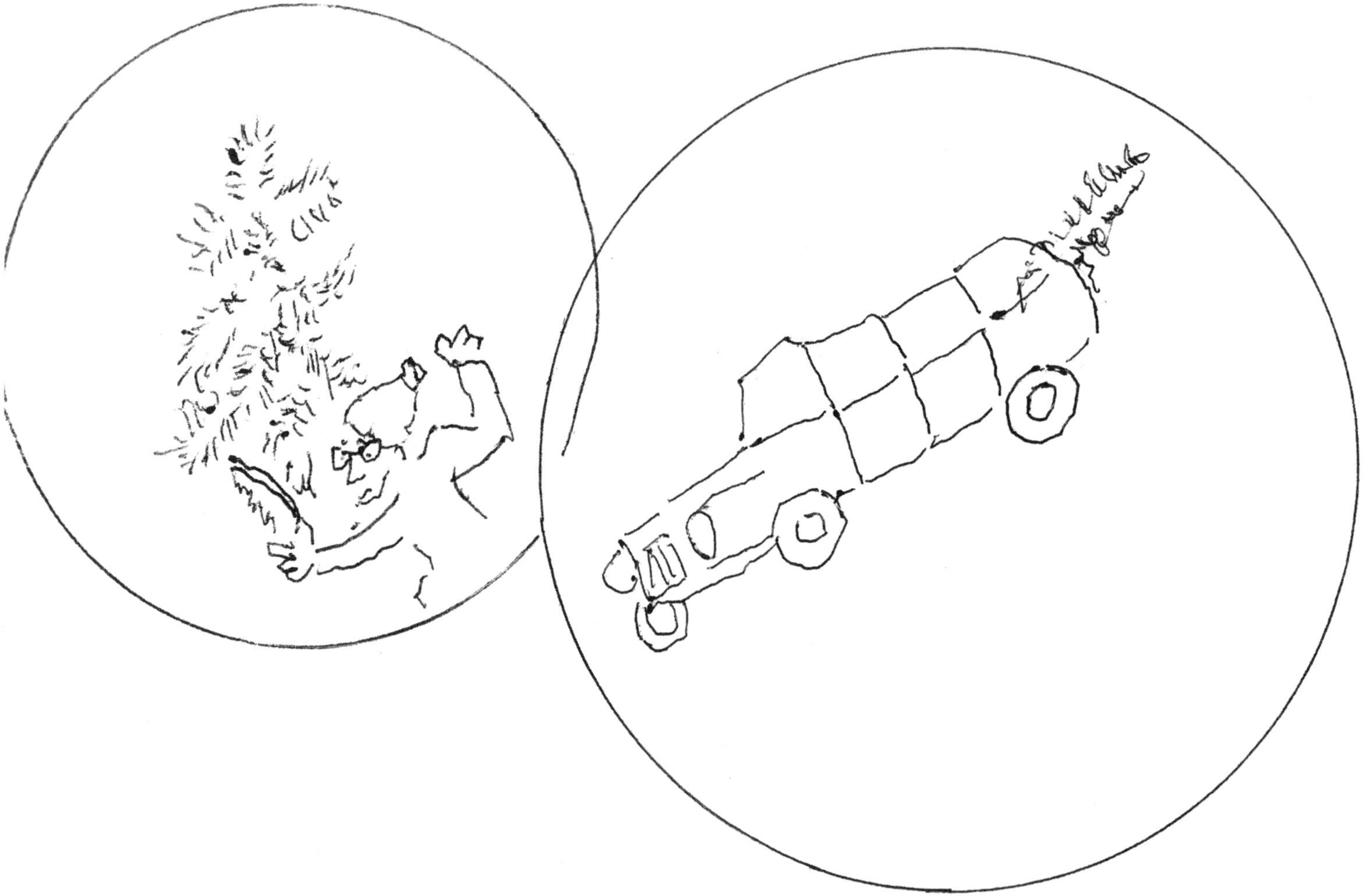

I experienced my first car accident when I was seven.

We had driven out to a forest reserve north and west of Calgary to harvest our annual Christmas tree. My family bumped along the old rutted forestry road till we arrived at the designated area. While my mother waited in the car and my father prepared dinner for us back at home, Nic, Liv, Ben, and I tramped, knee-deep in snow, through woods of Jack pine and fir until we identified a suitable tree. Nic, the eldest and thus entrusted with a saw, took the tree down. We loaded it onto a beat-up toboggan and dragged it back to the car. There, with the help of about a million yards of hemp rope and a series of complicated knots, we secured the tree to the roof of our old yellow station wagon and climbed back into the car, sticky with pinesap, and smelling of hot chocolate.

The sun dipped below the horizon and the skies, already overcast, lowered. Minutes after we left the forest reserve, snow began falling. Our afternoon activities had left me sleepy and I rested my head against the side panelling of the car door, the comforting hum of the motor shimmying through my body.

I was only barely awake when I spied a truck lumbering up the hill. It lurched, then jackknifed on the icy road. Moments later our car began a slow-motion spiral.

I could see the truck drawing close and my mother pumping the brakes. The vehicles made contact and I was jerked left as our car rebounded, then thrown forward as our car was struck from behind by another vehicle.

Now as I calm my mother, try but fail to make sense of her upset, coax her out of the washroom and get her dressed, as I encourage her to sit, and pour her a cup of coffee — I feel a familiar sense of vertigo, and a rising feeling of panic. Just beyond my direct line of vision a collision is looming.

And I know one thing. Everything is about to come undone.

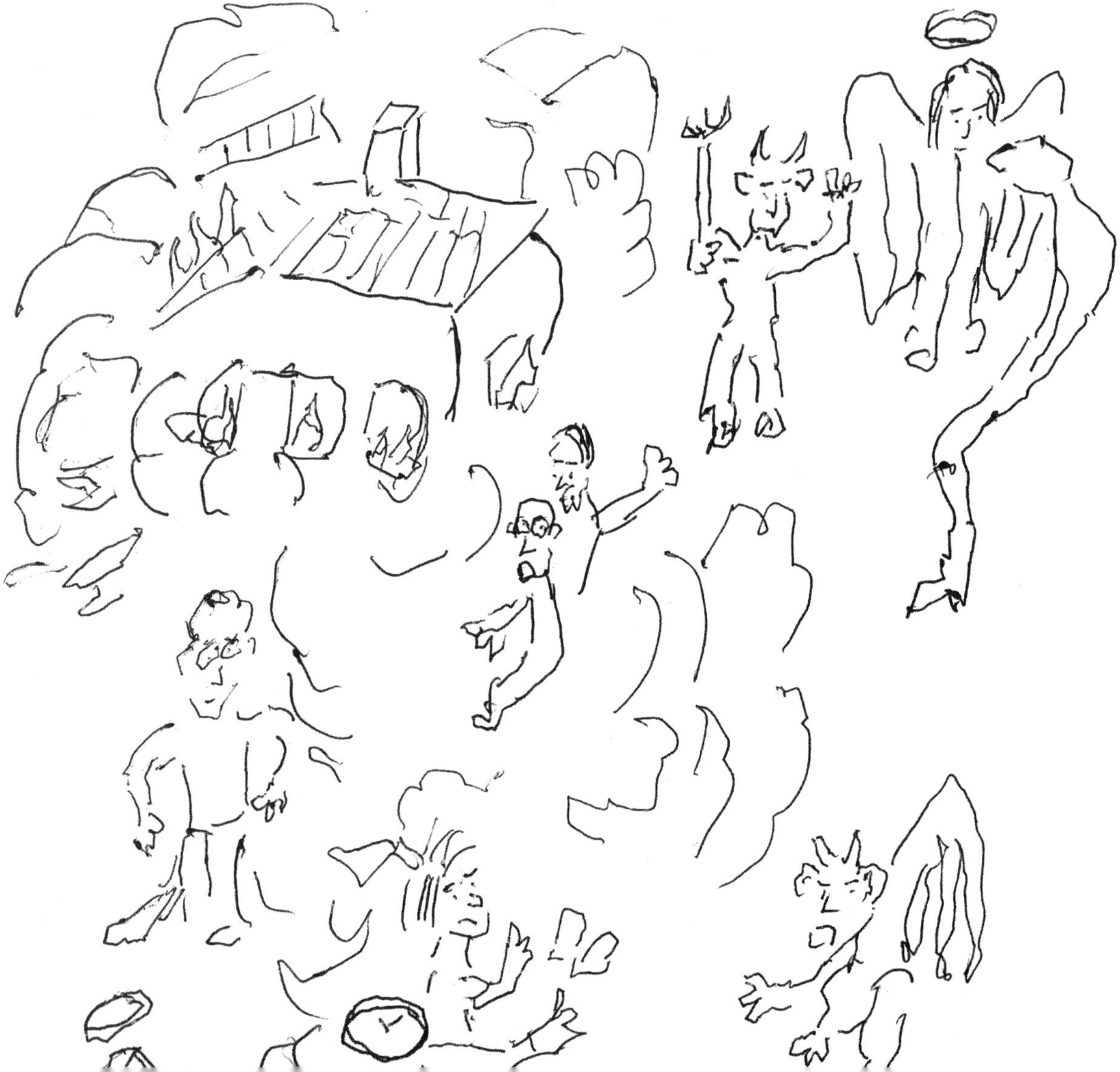

EVERY THING IS COMING APART

I stay with her until she feels more like herself, but as soon as I leave I email Nic. We've already held conversations about my mother's aging, her falls, and her increasing frailty. Nic has installed support railings in her washroom and an elevated toilet seat, and suggested that she get a call/alarm bracelet. But this latest situation seems like something new. He replies, letting me know that he'll visit Liv after work, then stop by Mom's.

I drive to the Loughheed to see how Liv is making out. He emerges slowly from his hospital room, feeling his way along the wall then grasping tabletops for support, as though navigating the heaving deck of an unsteady ship. When he sits at a table in the common area, it's with an abrupt, unexpected lurch.

I approach him, sit next to him, but he wears that same distant expression he bore the other day and says almost nothing. It's not clear if he even recognizes me. I try initiating conversation, but it never really catches. Eventually I stand, and tell him that Nic will be dropping by later and that I'll return the following day with Cheryl and my two daughters, Chandra and Miranda, then take my leave.

I wait at the reception desk to ask the psychiatric nurse on duty if anyone has yet determined what has happened to Liv. He tells me no, not yet.

I receive an email from Dr. Baxter telling me that the attending psychiatrist hopes to reintroduce clozapine. It turns out that hematology at the Foothills decided that, rather than selectively weaning Olivier off of one drug at a time, they would strip him of all his prescribed medications at once. They didn't see fit to tell either Liv or any other member of his family and apparently even his psychiatrist is only now finding out. This fracture in the chain of information has been a pattern I've seen repeated time and again over the years, but still I am astonished, once again, by the lack of cooperation between medical units, and the almost perverse, willful refusal to communicate clearly with psychiatric patients and their family.

In any case, the attending psychiatrist now believes that the drug that caused the previous low white blood count may have been a medication prescribed for gout, not clozapine. He'll put Liv back on the drug then closely monitor his blood work.

About three days into his stay at the hospital, Liv recognizes me and is able to sustain a conversation, but seems incredibly sad.

"I haven't been in the psych ward for years," he reflects wearily one afternoon. "I thought I was finished with all that." He gazes out at the snowy roofs of the city and the cottony steam trails rising from a thousand chimneys. "Who would have thought I would spend my sixtieth birthday here?"

I can understand his bewilderment and fatigue. It's been a long, long struggle for him and all of us, and schizophrenia is tireless.

I remember, when I first encountered it in our family, how frightened I was at its capacity to transform someone close and familiar into a stranger. I felt paralyzed by the disease.

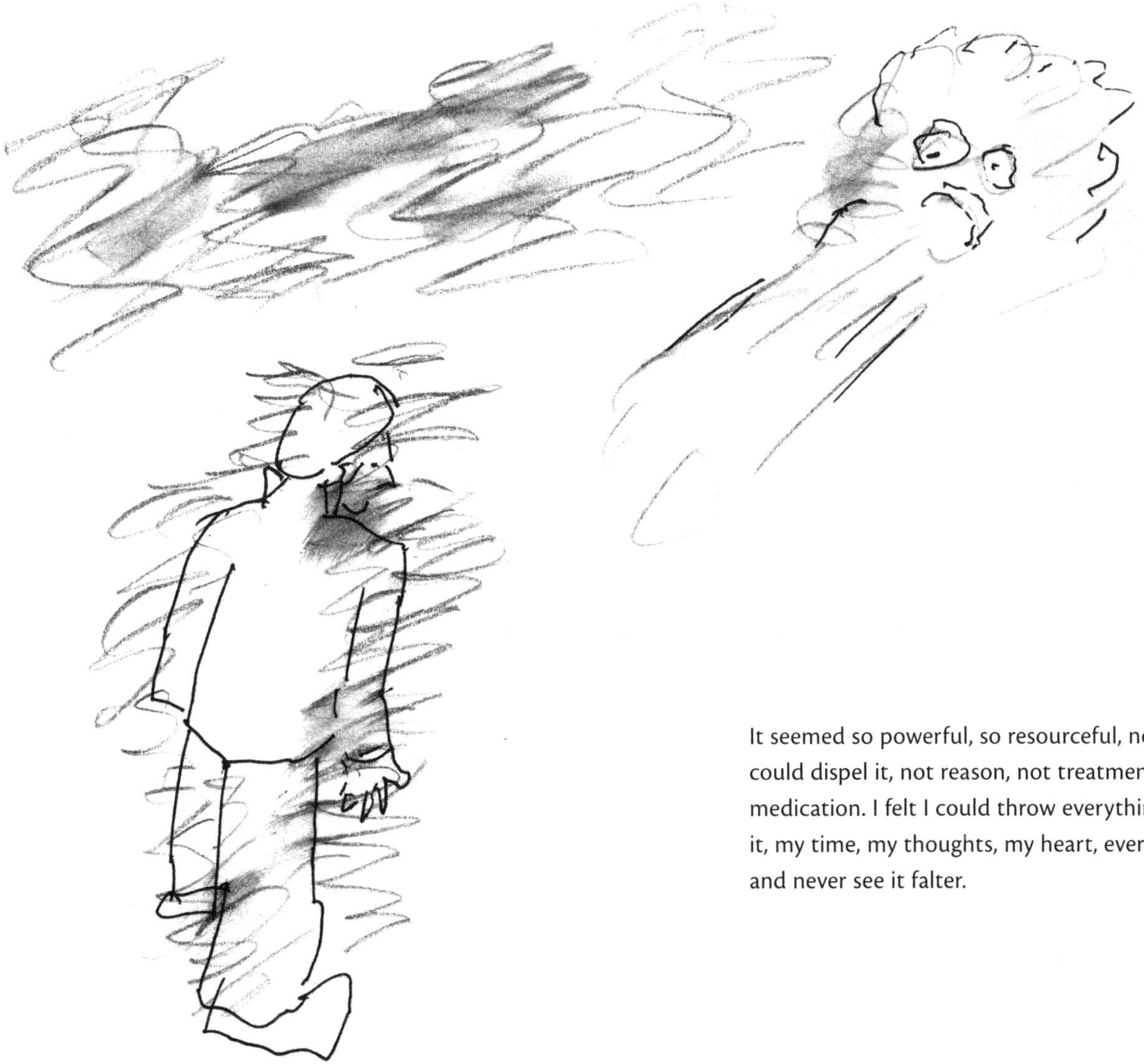

It seemed so powerful, so resourceful, nothing could dispel it, not reason, not treatment, not medication. I felt I could throw everything at it, my time, my thoughts, my heart, everything, and never see it falter.

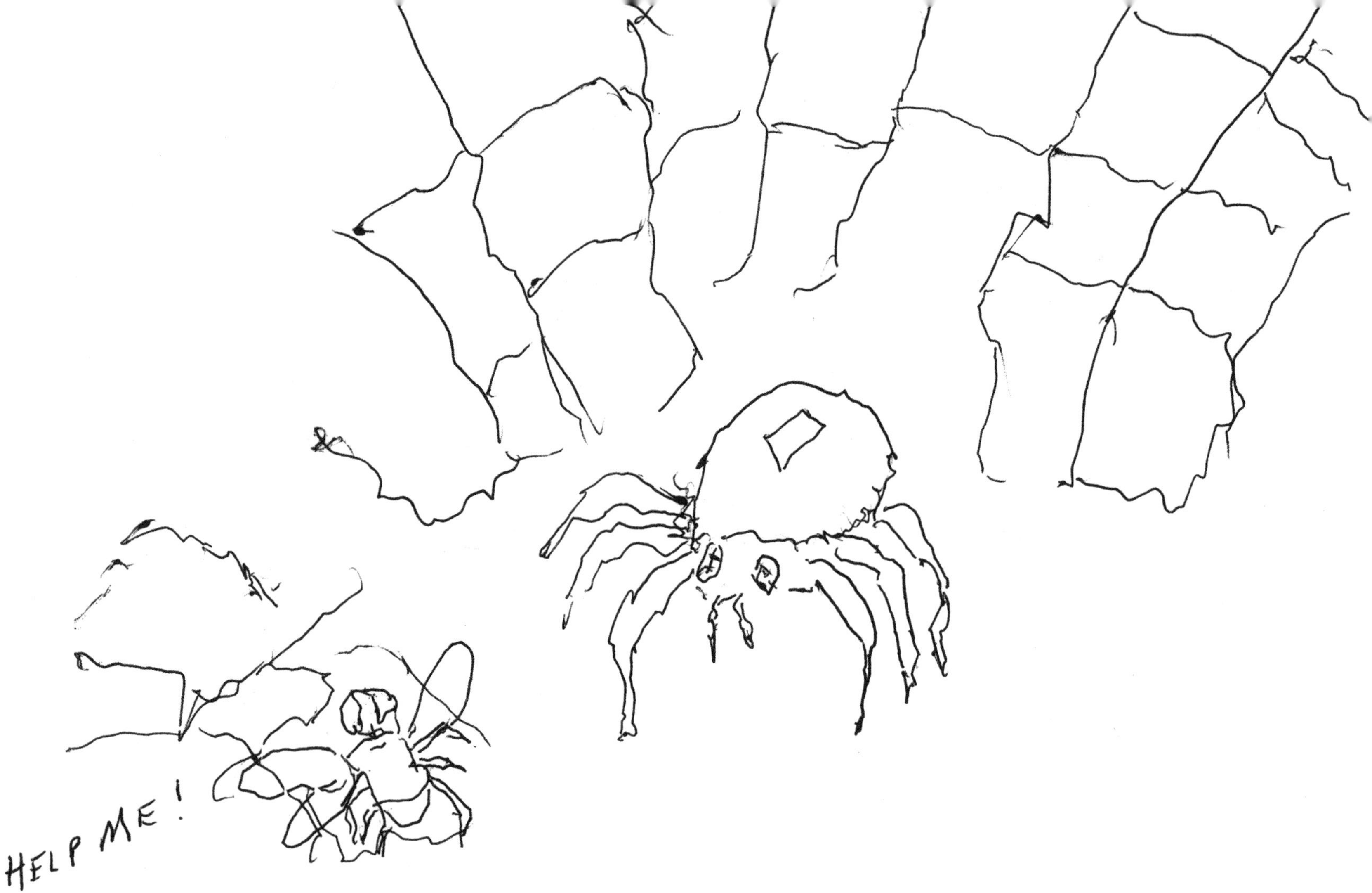
HELP ME!

Nic and I email back and forth trying to figure out what our next steps should be, but the problem is that everything about my mother and Olivier's living arrangements is so entirely intertwined. They co-own their apartment and split the monthly condominium fee. They share grocery expenses, utility expenses, daily household responsibilities, provide help and emotional support for one another in a thousand different ways. Liv is much more resilient now, but there was a time when his survival was uncertain, and the shared living arrangements were, without exaggeration, a lifesaver.

I've never much liked the term *caregiving*. It sounds too neat, too clear, too tidy. The impression it lends is that there exists this particular binary: someone who gives care, and someone who gets it.

In my experience that model is too simple. In reality, my mother provides financial and emotional support for my brother, certainly; at the same time Liv provides emotional support and companionship and physical help for her. My oldest brother, Nic, and I provide emotional support, assistance with groceries, communication with a variety of medical and government agencies, transportation to medical appointments around town, and emergency interventions when health situations arise, and it's the combination of all these intersecting efforts that allow everyone to carry on. What we provide is less a direct give-and-get than it is an interconnected network of care, like a spider's web.

But it isn't pretty. The truth is that it more closely resembles the flawed, wonky structures generated by the spiders given LSD during lab experiments in the sixties than the glorious, dew-dappled symmetry you might spy hanging from some branches on an early morning walk. This web is fashioned as much from good intentions and competencies as is from compensations, mistakes, and frailties. It sustains and supports, but only barely. Snap a single thread and everything tumbles away.

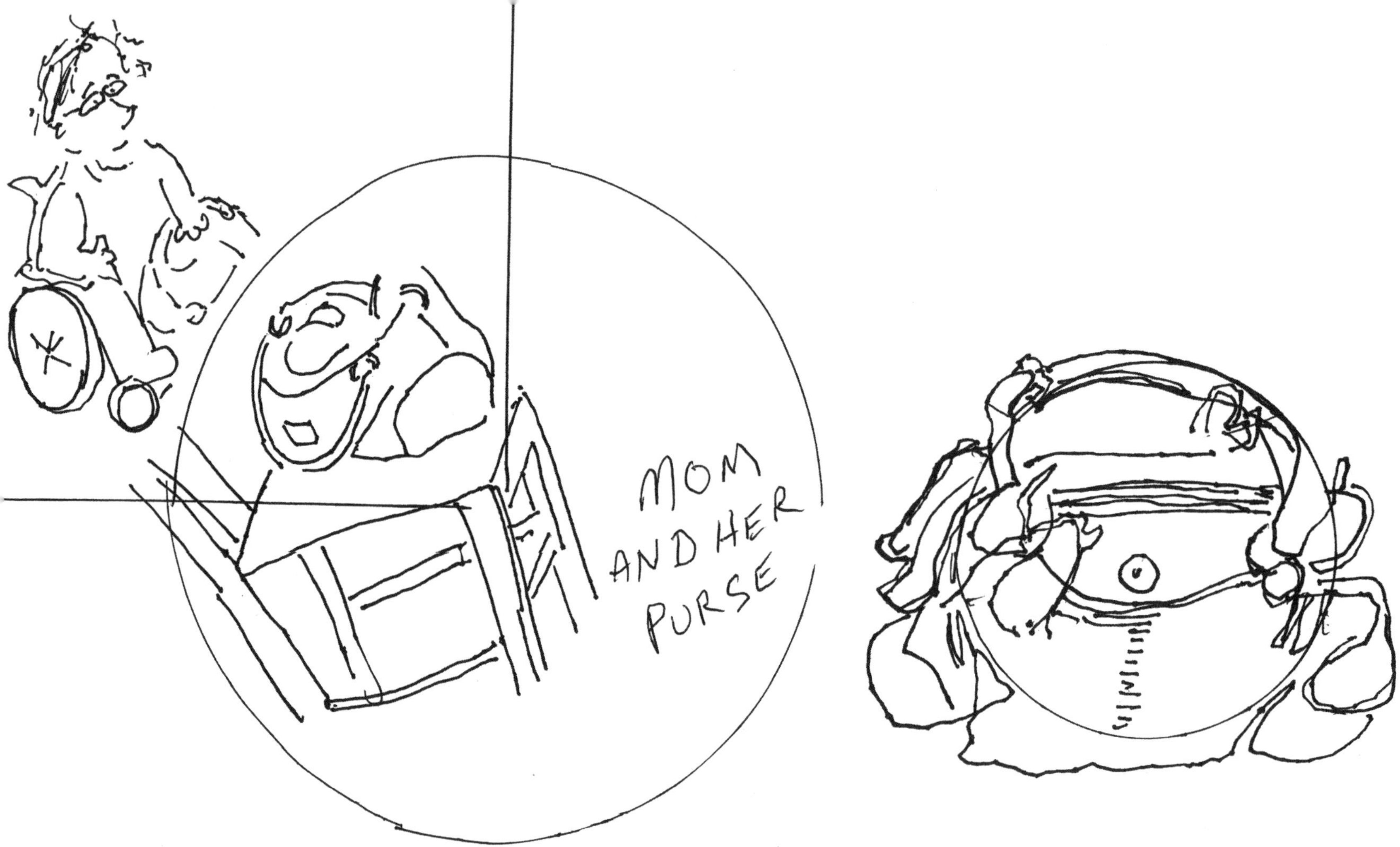
MOM
AND HER
PURSE

Liv continues to improve at the hospital. Bit by bit he grows more able to express himself again, participates in group therapy, and is permitted to go off-ward for coffee with visitors. A few days later, he receives a trial weekend pass. He buses home, is able to function much as he did before, then returns to the psychiatric ward Sunday night.

The following Monday he's fully discharged. I drive to the hospital to pick him up, he quietly collects his things, and I take him to the apartment. Mom is relieved to have him back — but things have changed. Whether it is the confusion and anxiety of having Olivier fall ill so quickly, or whether it has been the stress of living alone, from this point on, my mother's quirks escalate.

A few weeks after Liv has returned home, he calls me from a neighbour's and asks if I can come by the apartment and figure out why their phone isn't working. I drive over, pick up their receiver, and listen. There's no dial tone. I hang up, check to see if the phone is plugged in, then ask Liv if they have paid the bills.

He says he doesn't know.

I ask Mom. She says she doesn't know.

"Well," I ask, confused, "how have the bills been paid in the past?"

Neither of them answer.

"Where are they kept?" I ask.

Mom tells me she collects them in her purse.

"Can I have a look?" I ask.

She hands me her purse, and I rifle through it. Deep in one side pocket there's a thick stack of envelopes, maybe thirty, most unopened. One of them is lined in red, a final notice.

"This is a notice to disconnect," I tell her. "Why haven't you opened it?" She stares at me.

I call from my cell phone, restore telephone service by paying with my credit card, and arrange to have the bill paid automatically at the end of each month.

I hang up, withdraw the remaining bills from Mom's purse, and go through them. They're all in arrears: gas, electric, cable TV. I ask why she didn't open them? She doesn't know. Didn't she understand, I demand, that these would have to be paid? She just returns my stare. I tell her that I'm going to arrange for all of the bills to be debited automatically from her account.

That's the short-term solution, but we are going to have to go to the bank and make some changes so that I can help manage her financial affairs. Good, she says, and reaches for a crossword puzzle book.

A couple of days later I swing by to pick Mom up for our appointment at the bank. Although she was initially grateful that I offered to manage her bills, she now appears to have forgotten the reason why I made that offer. Instead, she views this transfer of responsibility as a favour she's doing me. She says if I need money to just let her know. I don't need her money, I remind her, I just need to know that her bills are getting paid.

As we're leaving I offer to help her carry her very heavy purse, but she snatches it from my grasp. She's suddenly become particularly protective of it, and will inform anyone who will listen that it contains "her entire life."

While waiting in the bank's lobby to be seen by the bank manager, I become aware of a lingering, powerfully unpleasant odour. The longer we wait, the more certain I become that the smell is coming from my mother, and that everyone in the bank can detect it as well. A few months past, the garburator at the apartment had jammed and then flooded. Mom had asked me to recommend a plumber, but even after the plumber came and went and the problem was fixed, the smell lingered on. Now that smell has followed us into the bank.

A receptionist finally approaches, glances at my mother, and frowns briefly, then guides us through a hallway to an office, where we squeeze into tiny seats at the manager's majestic desk.

I explain that my mother has experienced difficulty making payments on time, and we have agreed that the solution is for me to help out. The manager seems sympathetic — I imagine that he sees this sort of thing often. He suggests we establish a General Power of Attorney, and provides us with the forms to sign.

On the drive back to the apartment I tell Mom she may want to dispose of her Depend undergarments more frequently, and ensure that Liv take them promptly to the waste station. She nods.

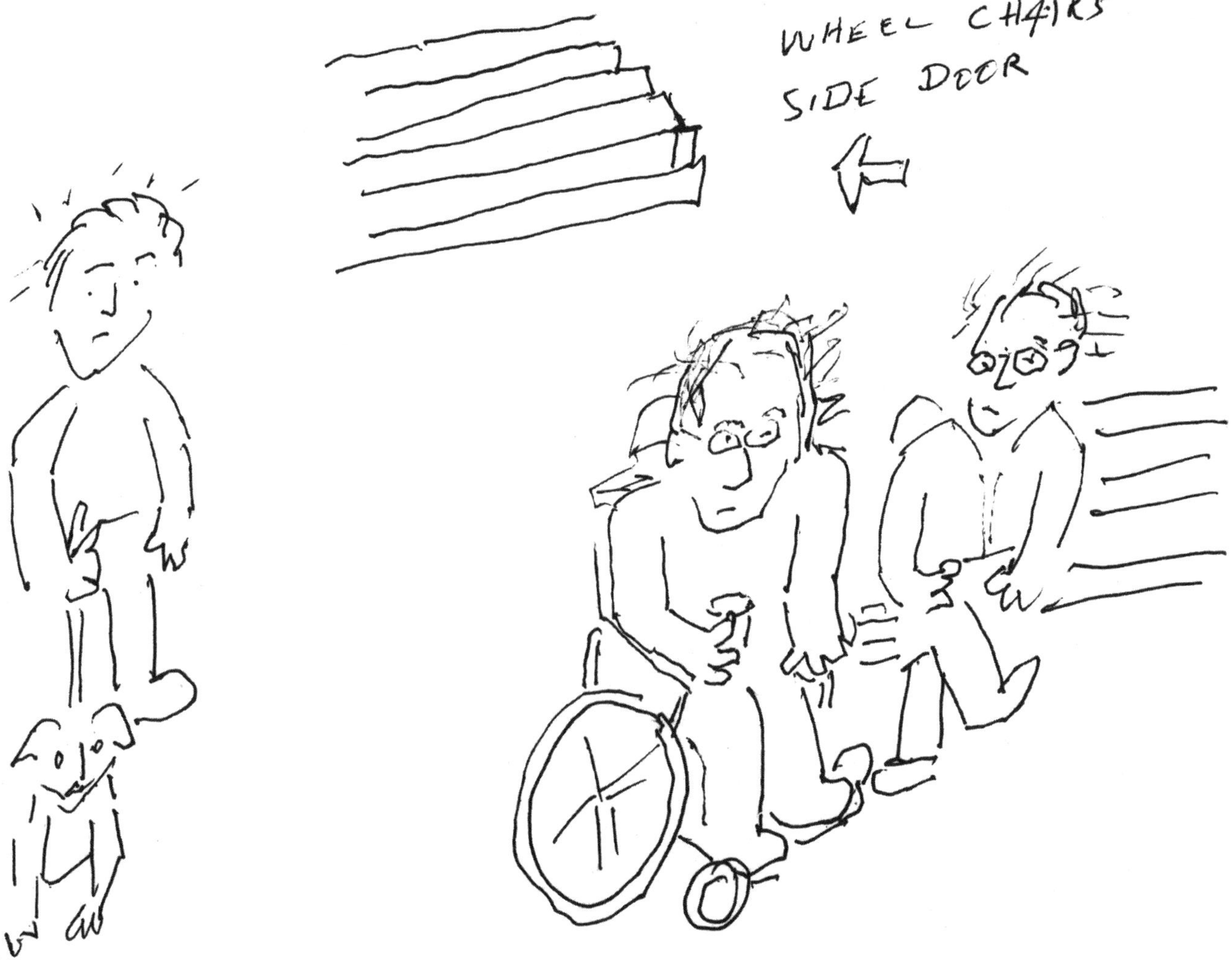
WHEEL CHAIRS
SIDE DOOR

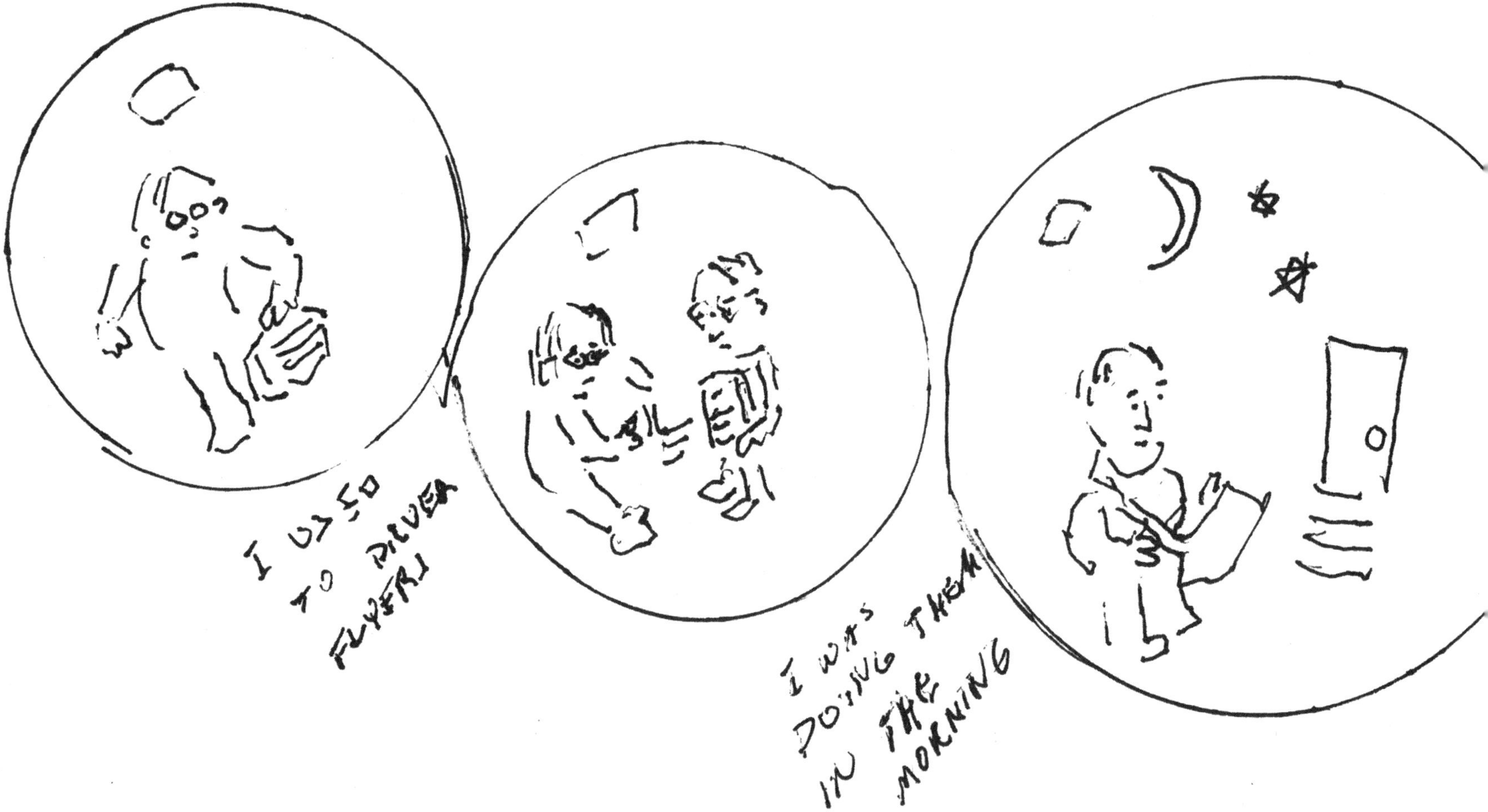
I USED TO DIVER FLYERS
I WAS DOING THEM IN THE MORNING

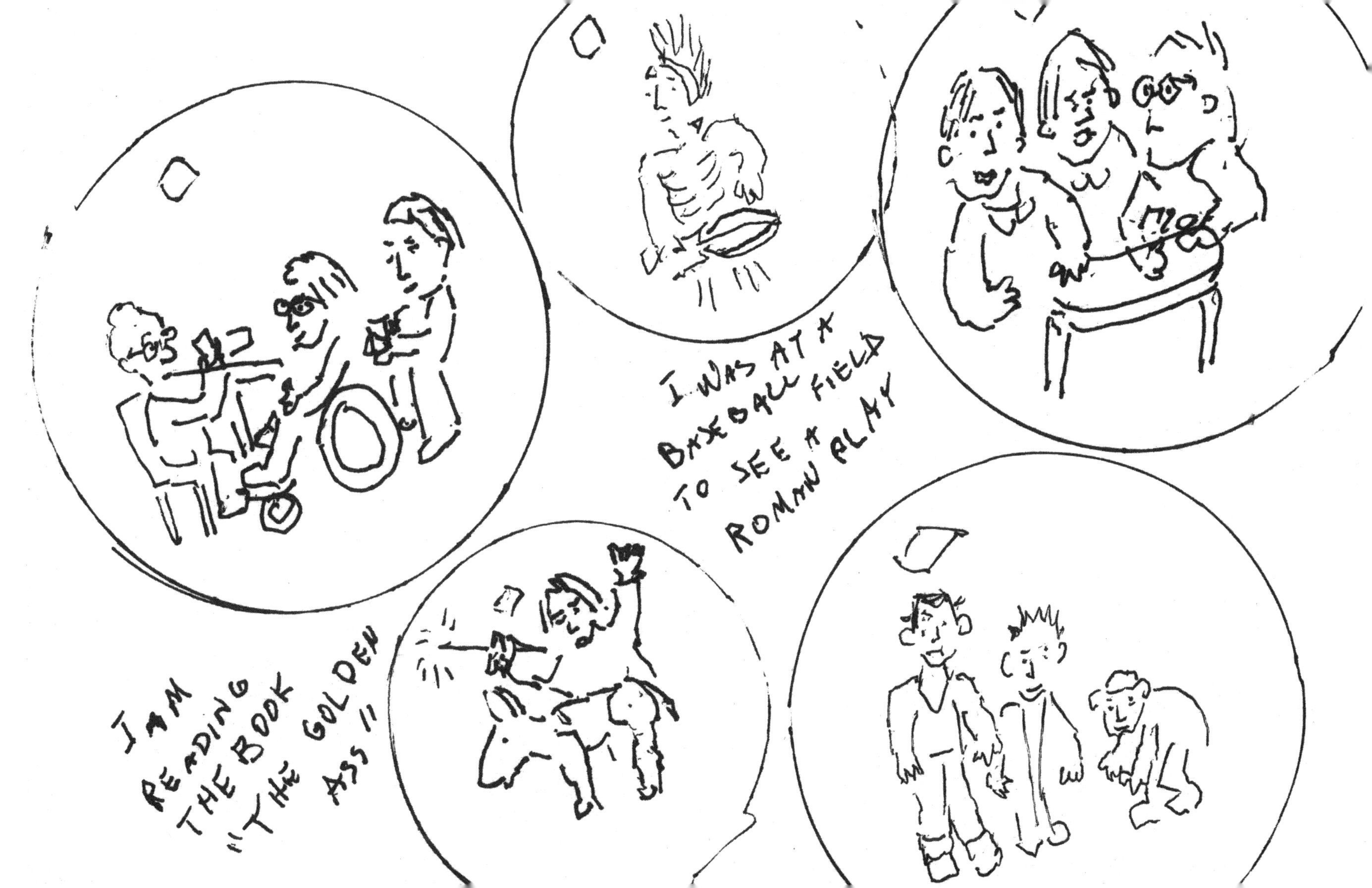
I WAS AT A BASEBALL FIELD TO SEE A ROMAN PLAY
I AM READING THE BOOK "THE GOLDEN ASS"

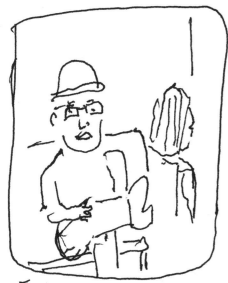

I GOT ON THE BUS ON
WRONG SIDE OF THE
STREET SO I HAD TO
GO TO THE END OF LINE
AND BACK

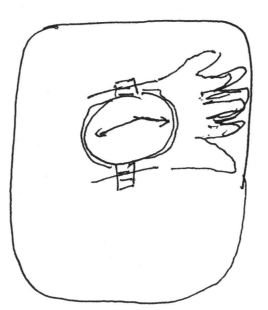

I WAS WORRIED ABOUT
MEETING MOM AT THE
COOP AT 2:00.

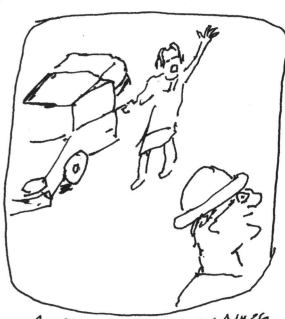

AS I WAS ENTERING
CROWFOOT COOP, MOM
CALLED TO ME.

I enroll in an online course called "Caring for People with Psychosis and Schizophrenia" offered by King's College London. The four-week course features videos, articles, and lectures. Liv's recent setbacks and my mother's confusion have flung me into the farthest deep end of the pool and I'm hoping the course will provide me with new flotation devices.

Each day I check the website, review my course materials, complete tests, and participate in the chat room. It's comforting to know that others have experienced the same things I have and feel just as inadequate.

A quote from one of the professors of psychiatric research, Sir Robin Murray, resonates with me. *"There is the professional team who can help the patient. But, of course, the important thing is for the patient to have help and support in the community. And this is where the family is most important. People who have the best outlook are those who have supportive family. And, of course, it's important for psychiatrists and psychologists to involve the patient and the patient's relatives in decisions. I would say to families, you should keep pushing and ensure that your relative does have access to the best pharmacological treatment, the best psychological treatment, that they get some social help, and that they keep busy. The worst thing is to be staring at the wall, hallucinating."*

I am both encouraged and disheartened by this statement. If, as seems to be the case, families have such a significant role to play in assisting with treatment, why is so little effort made to include or support families at an institutional level? Why is it that whenever I accompany Liv to the hospital I'm made to feel like I'm crashing a party to which I wasn't invited?

Dr. Murray also confirms that I'm not alone in my perception that there is a disjunction between the psychiatric level of care and the physical health services — it's a worldwide phenomenon:

"One of the major concerns carers had about current care planning was that service users' physical health needs were not being met alongside their mental illness. In some cases, they felt that physical illnesses were entirely omitted from current care plans, and this reflected a similar problem in wider health records, whereby mental illness was often not recorded on physical health records. This was often attributed to a lack of connection between mental and physical health services, and became particularly problematic when service users were hospitalized in a crisis, for either their mental or physical health problem."

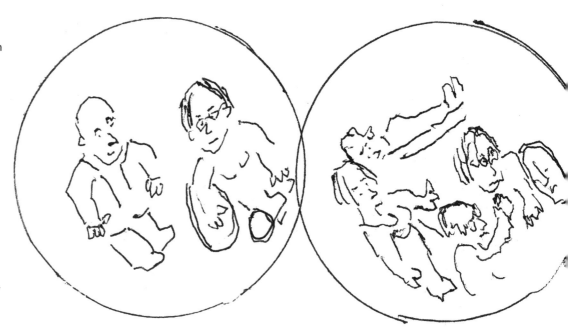

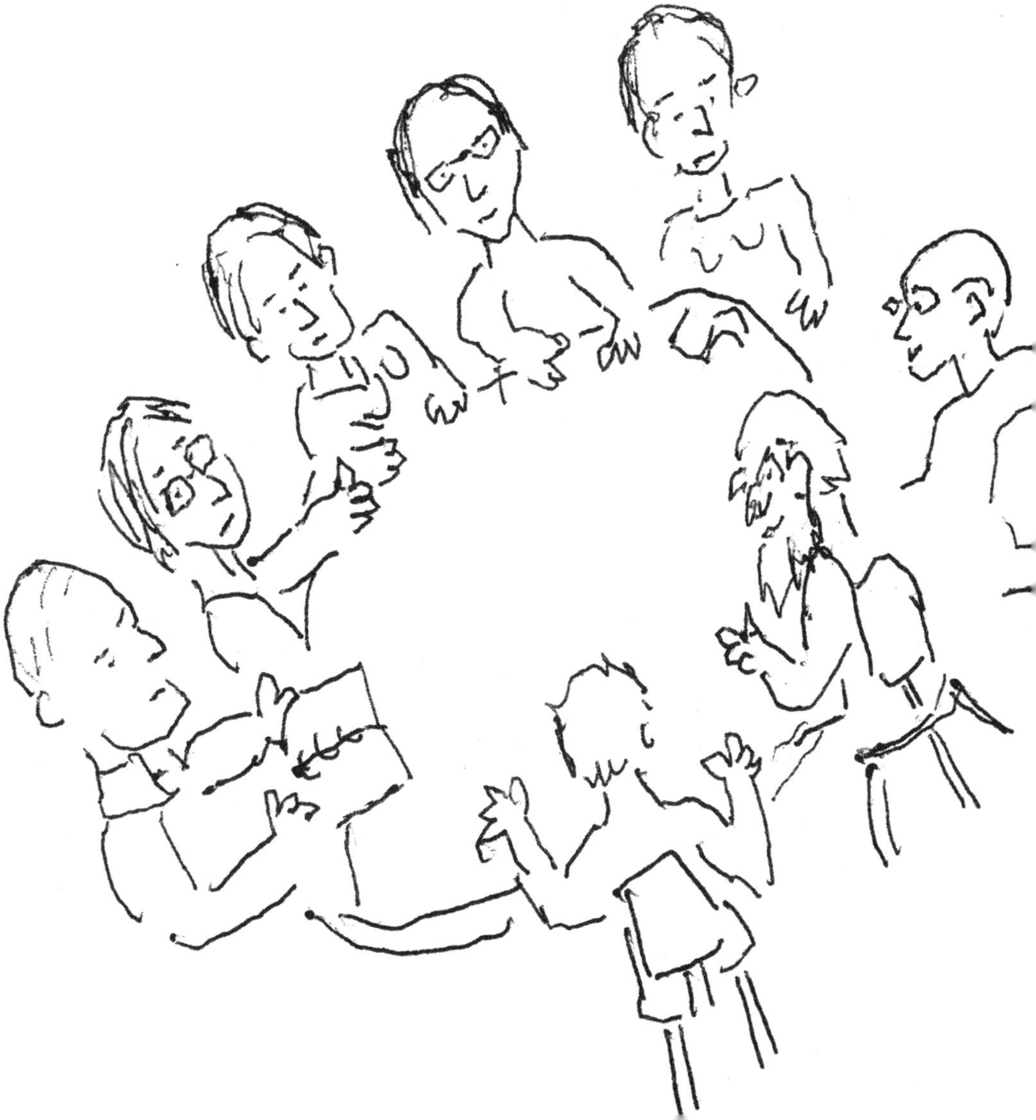

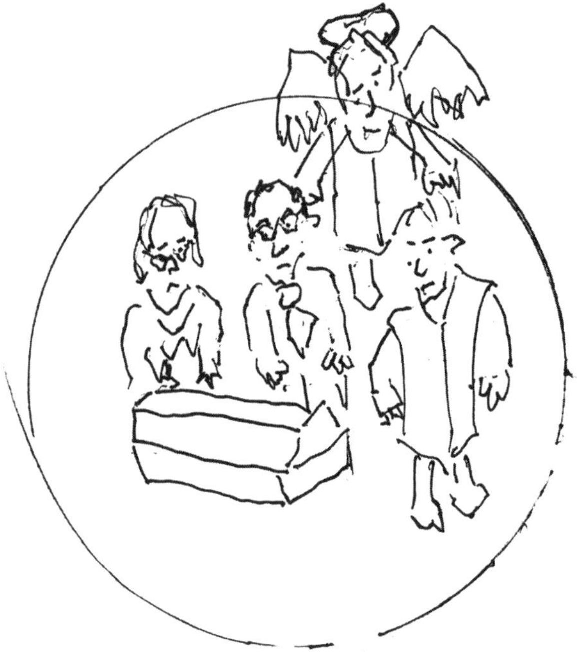

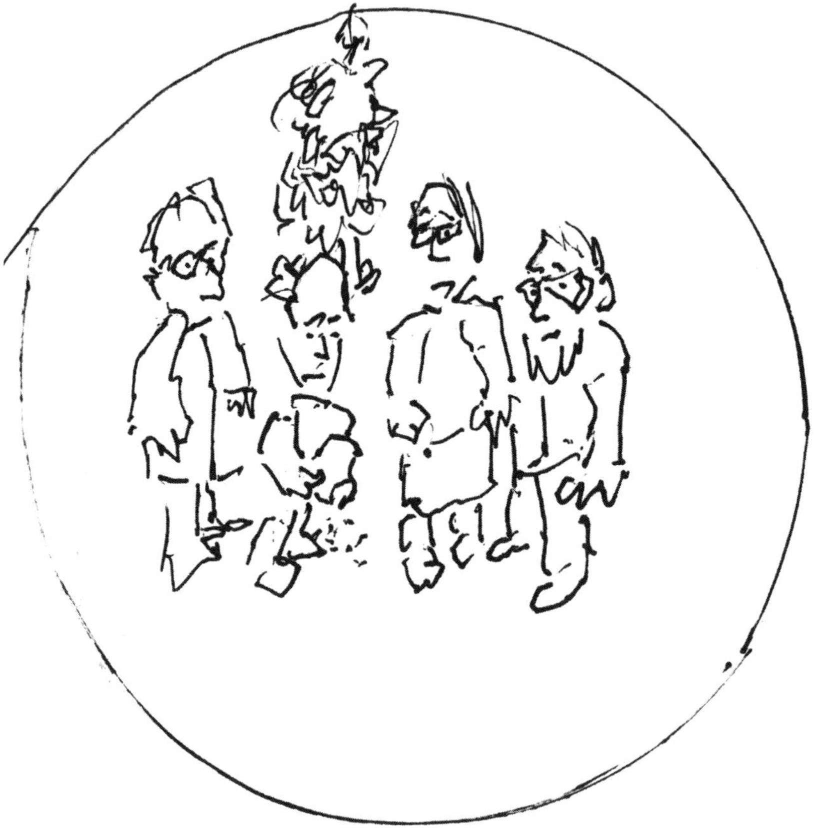

My father discovered my younger brother's body.

The way it happened was that Ben didn't show up for his group therapy one afternoon. His psychiatrist called my mother to express his concern and my mother phoned around, hoping to learn where Ben had gone. She discovered from one of his high school friends that he had purchased a gun. Ben, in his most paranoid moments, had focused his anger on Olivier, and Mom panicked. Convinced that Ben had taken his gun and gone after Olivier, she ran to the car and drove to Olivier's apartment, hoping to intercept Ben.

The house was silent, everyone believing it to be empty. Dad descended into the basement to double-check and found the overhead bulbs had burnt out. In the shadows of the basement he spied the partial outline of a solitary figure reclining in a chair. He called out. Not receiving an answer, he approached the figure, touched it, and withdrew a hand covered in blood.

My father shared that memory with me only months before he passed away in 1988, and it was clear, a decade after my younger brother's death, that he remained haunted by it. He told me that he felt he'd failed not only Ben but all his surviving sons.

People tend to think of suicide as a solitary act, but it's not. Suicide is transformative, changing everything it touches – family relationships, family traditions, exchanges between individuals, the ways that you look at people, the ways you look at life. The positively energized atoms of your previous life are expunged and replaced with other atoms fashioned of clay and coal dust. You wake one morning and find you are a different person. The guilt my mother bore reshaped her. Liv's diagnosis seemed a confirmation of all her suspicions of inadequacy. She grew more guarded, detected in every comment a criticism of her family, or of her ability to provide care, or both.
She determined never to make a mistake again, never to fail to read the signs. She'd lost one son to schizophrenia; she wouldn't lose another.

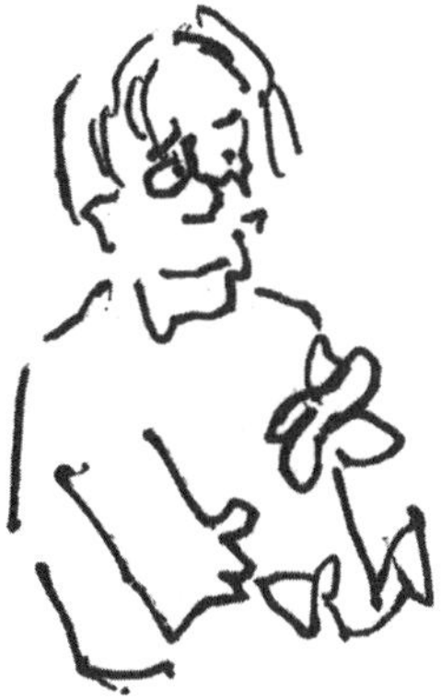

I'm in my office at the University of Calgary marking papers when my mother calls.

"Clem? Help! I've fallen." Her voice on the other end of the line is shrill and edged with panic.

"Where are you?" I ask.

"At home! I've been lying on the floor for hours. I dragged myself to the table and knocked the phone over. Help, help, help!"

"Are you bleeding?" I interrupt. "Have you broken anything? Should I call an ambulance?"

"No, I just can't get up," she gasps. "Help! Help—"

"Mom!" I interrupt again. "Shouldn't I get a paramedic for you?"

"No!" she wails. "Just come as quick as you can."

"It'll take me twenty minutes to half an hour to get there."

"Fine. Hurry!"

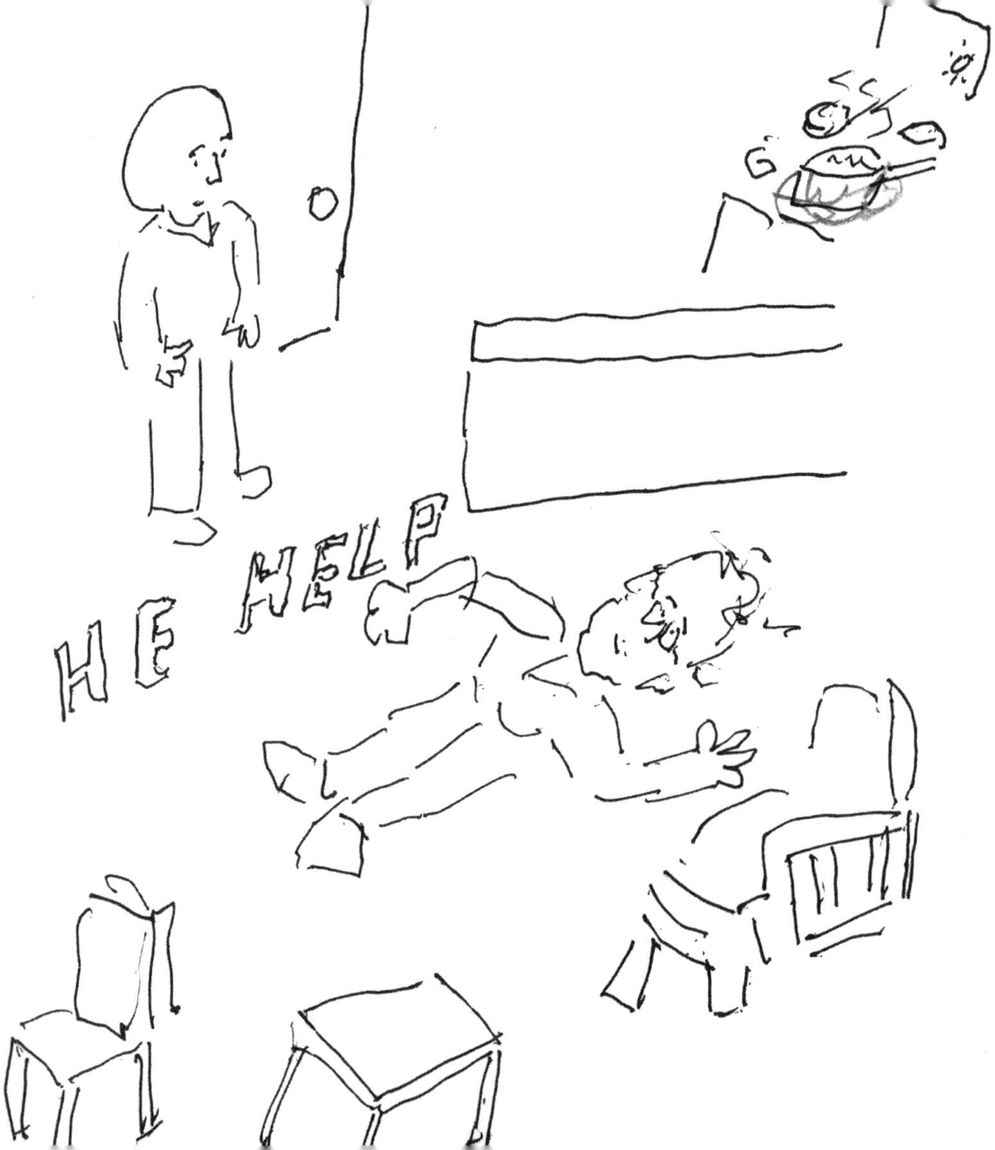
HE HELP

I send a text cancelling my upcoming grad seminar, and hurry to my car.

When I enter the condominium, I find her lying on the floor, the coffee table overturned.

"Is anything sprained or broken?" I ask, kneeling and placing a hand on her shoulder.

She shakes her head. "No. Just set me back up in my chair."

I rock back on my heels and consider the situation. There's no easy way to do it — her arms have so little muscle tone that she can't offer any support. I reach around her, brace my legs, and strain to lift her — she may not be a large woman but she's dead weight. Suddenly she shrieks. I freeze and break into a sweat.

"Mom, what's wrong?" I shout, trying to cut through her panic, but she just keeps screaming, shrill, high-pitched, inarticulate.

I can't tell if I'm compressing a broken bone or pinching an internal injury or just frightening her, and she is unable to provide me with any clues. I don't feel I can safely set her back down on the floor, so I grit my teeth and continue lifting. As gently as I can, I place her in her chair. She stops screaming and closes her eyes in relief.

In the silence that follows, I upright the coffee table, replace the telephone to its original position, lift her walker, and stand it next to the chair. The palms of my hands are sweating and I wipe them against my jeans.

I pour and then bring her a glass of water, which she gratefully accepts and quickly drains. I ask if she is sure she is okay — she nods. Is she certain I shouldn't take her to the hospital? No, she's feeling better now. She'll be fine if

I just leave her with another glass of water and a biscuit.

Later, when I speak with Liv about her fall, he says that since he's returned home there have been a half dozen nights when he's had to help her up after she's taken a tumble on her way to the washroom.

I hang up the phone, and close my eyes. Just last night, in the online discussion for my caregiving course, I read a comment from a parent in Ireland: *"My biggest worry is also what will happen when I die. Who will look after my son? Some practical advice on preparing for this inevitability would be extremely helpful."*

Another member of the group had replied:

"The anxiety is there on the other side too! My parents are getting elderly and I'm really anxious about how I'll cope without them."

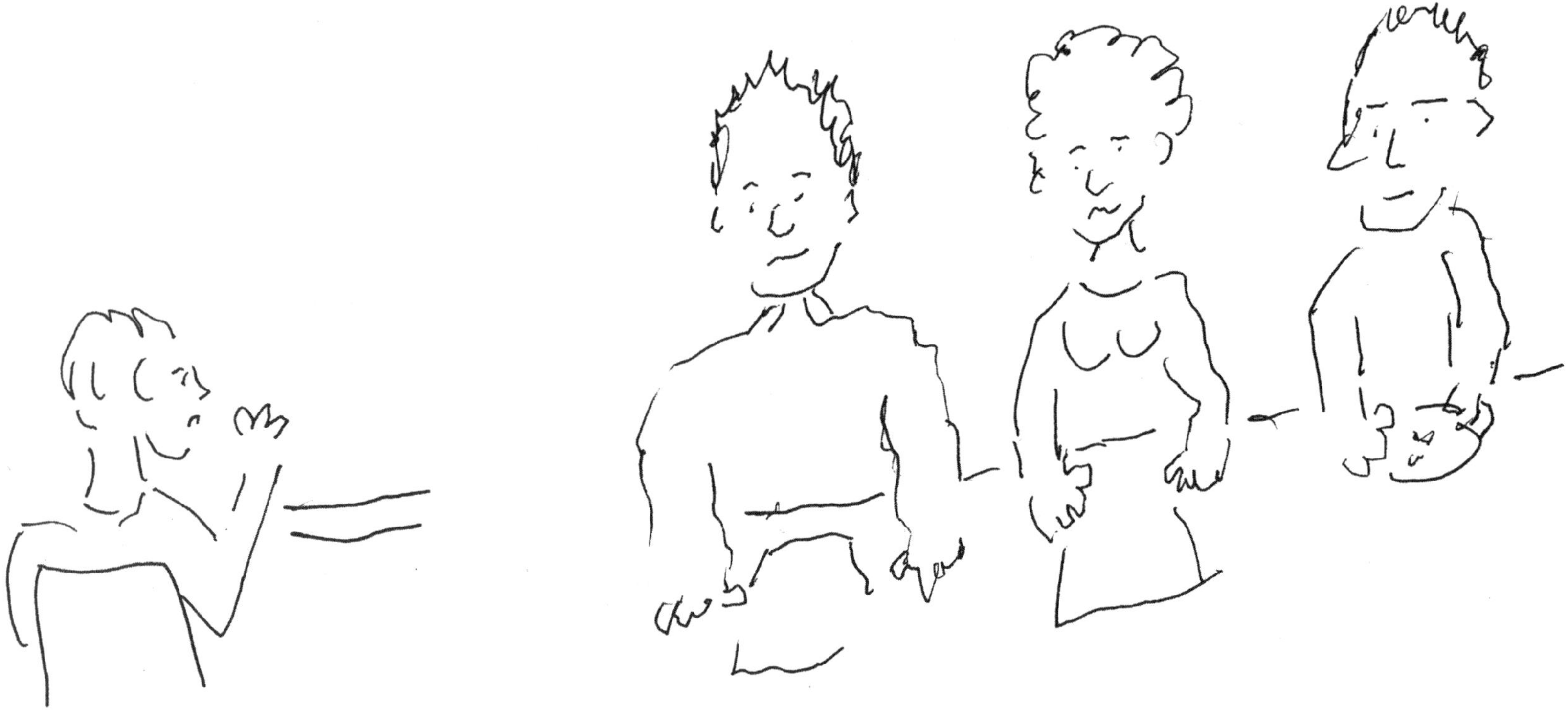

The day after my mother's fall, Nic and I book an appointment with a social worker to explore our options. I park the car in the shade of a gnarled poplar that has forced its way up through the cracked, lumpy parking lot. The seniors' social services office is located next to the parking lot, in what was once an old school, but is now host to a variety of social agencies clustered under the one roof.

Our counsellor is a middle-aged woman with flushed cheeks and an air of being slightly behind in her schedule. Her office is compact, barely able to accommodate her desk and lamp, and I wonder what this space might have been when it was part of a school — perhaps the mop room. She drags in a chair from the foyer, crams it beside the other, and we crowd knee to knee around her desk.

Dispensing with any small talk, she shoves a fistful of brochures at us. "You'll need these," she says, "read them." Her tone is that of someone delivering a prepared talk — and I suppose she is. She probably meets with people like my brother and me a dozen times a week.

"How old is your mother and how frail?" she asks, pushing her glasses up her nose with an air of getting down to business. It will be essential for our mother to be assessed for her mental and physical competencies. That assessment will provide the medical authorities with the information necessary to decide which level of care is most appropriate: home care or a placement at a facility. And it can take months to years, she tells us — *months to years* — to get into an assisted living facility. So, if there is even a remote chance that this may become an eventuality, we should begin preparations immediately.

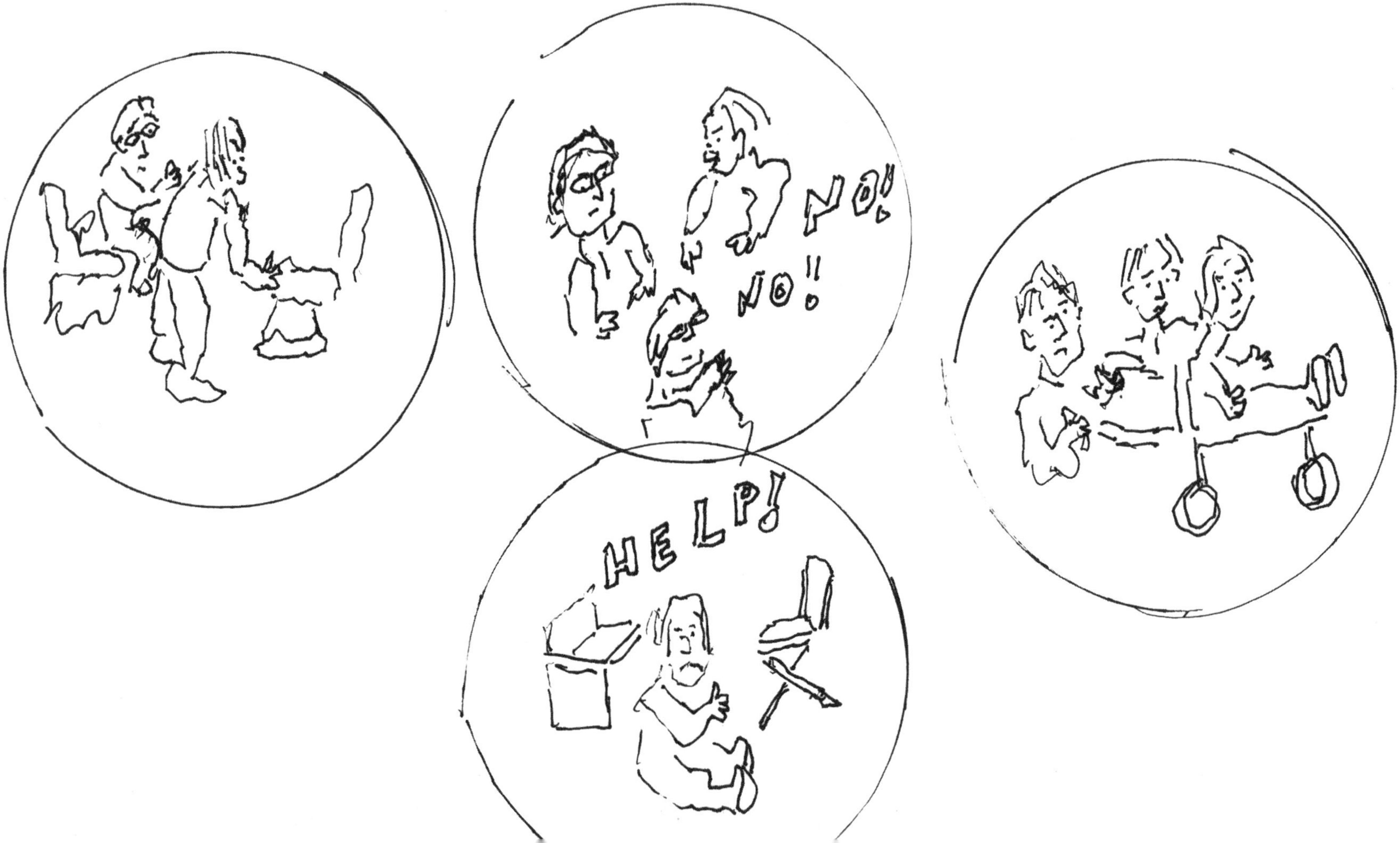
NO!
NO!!
HELP!

But Nic and I have already tested those waters and our mother has made it clear that she has no interest in assisted living. She wants to age in place, she insists, and when she dies, it's to be in her bed.

Nevertheless, Nic schedules and then accompanies Mom to an assessment with her long-time family doctor. Nic describes Mom's falls, her confusion, her inability to care for herself. The GP performs a brief and rather perfunctory evaluation. He asks Mom how she feels. She allows that old age is a trial. He administers a memory test, asking her to recollect a series of facts in sequence. When later required to confirm those facts, she remembers some, forgets others, and in the end her doctor simply writes up an assessment stating that she demonstrates some "age-appropriate memory loss" and should be able to cope in her home. That's it.

My heart drops when Nic gives me the note to read.

"Well," I say, handing it back to Nic. "That's no good. One of these times she'll fall and it will be serious."

"It could have been serious the last time," he observes glumly. "She cut her forehead. She could have broken her collarbone."

"Or she'll set fire to the condominium." I'm thinking of the pot she burned cooking porridge two days ago.

Our next option is to explore home care, which requires another assessment, this time in her home.

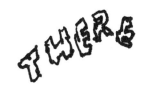

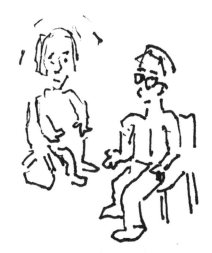

We prepare Mom for the interview, but she's not inclined to make the process easy. She greets the home care supervisor coldly and treats every question as either irrelevant or humiliating.

"Can I *cook*?" she repeats, rolling her eyes. "Of course I can *cook*! I've been cooking since I could reach the stovetop! Can I *look after myself*? I've been looking after myself since before you were born!"

The situation isn't helped by the fact that she can't actually hear the supervisor. She places a hand aside her ear, grimaces, and shouts "What?" after every second sentence.

The supervisor leans in close and shouts into my mother's face. "Do you pee frequently?" she hollers. "Can you clean after yourself?"

This allows her to be heard but isn't much of an improvement. My mother bristles at the invasion the proximity represents, and feels insulted by the elementary vocabulary employed. "Do you think I'm a *baby*?" she snaps.

"No—"

"Do you think I'm *stupid*?"

Still, at the conclusion of the meeting my mother agrees — grudgingly, very grudgingly — to accept help. Staff will arrive every two days to tidy, give my mother a hand with her shower, and prepare a lunch. A schedule is posted on the fridge.

Before she leaves, the supervisor asks if we wish to have my mother placed on the wait-list for assisted living. She repeats the familiar refrain: that it takes a considerable time to get the forms processed, and then additional time to actually be offered a placement, that you don't necessarily have to accept a placement once it's offered. My mother, surprisingly, and perhaps only because she's tired of arguing, agrees.

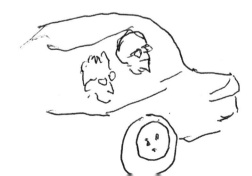

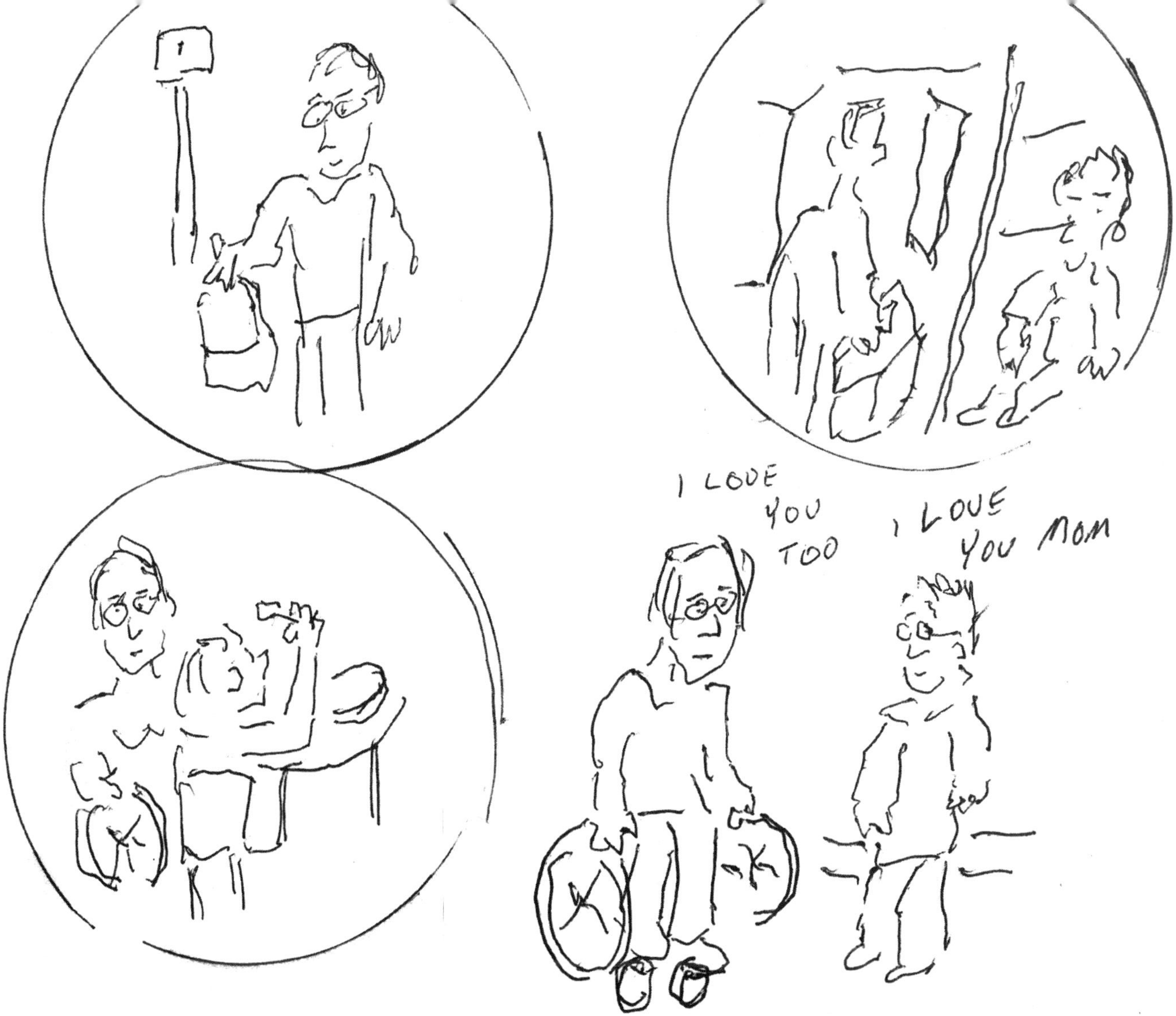
I LOVE YOU MOM
I LOVE YOU TOO

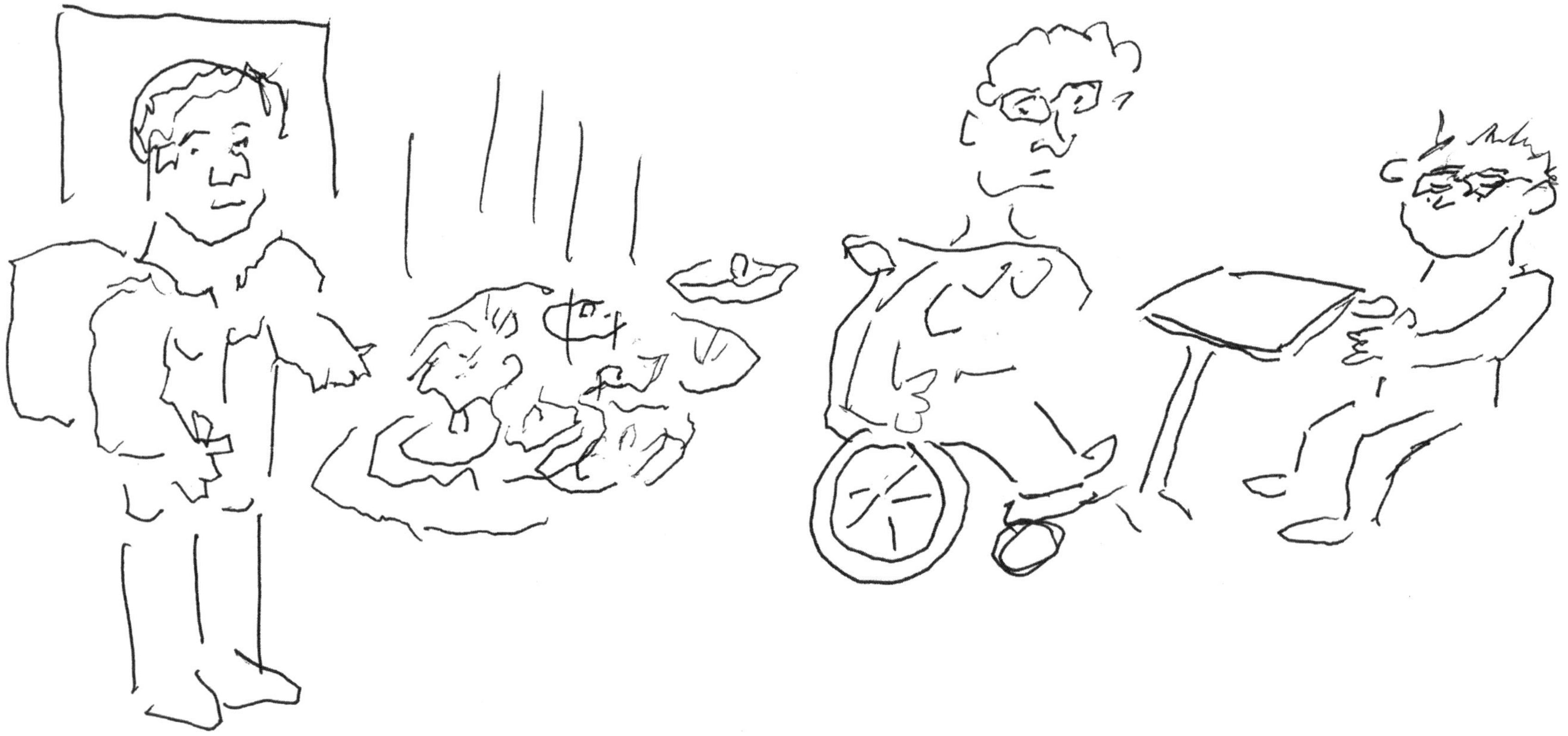

Home care commences and is an immediate disaster. A young man appears at our mother's door, announcing he's come to administer the shower. Mom responds with fury. She chases him out, shouting as he goes, and phones Nic to ask *what were we thinking*? Did we mistakenly believe her to be the kind of woman that preferred to be *scrubbed by a boy*? If this is the kind of *help* she can expect, she fumes, we can cancel it right away. We call home care. They apologize, assure us it was all a mistake and will be corrected.

Problems arise from the scheduling. My mother wakes early — usually by five — but home care can't guarantee that anyone will arrive before nine. My mother balks at getting dressed and ready for her day, only to have to undress and restart her day with a shower four hours later. Home care arranges for staff to drop by in the afternoon instead, but they show up late. My mother, fanatical about punctuality, is driven to distraction.

Visitors have to be buzzed into my mother's condo. Home care representatives routinely arrive, lean on the buzzer, get no response, and depart. My mother claims not to hear the buzzer. We install a lockbox at the main entrance so that the home care workers can let themselves in, but this means they often startle my hard-of-hearing mother.

Most of my mother's close friends have passed away, so my mother complains that the hours drag by. Nic arranges for home care to have her picked up and taken to a social gathering with other seniors. She attends once, then refuses to go again, informing us that the programming — mostly playing Monopoly and other board games — is designed for youngsters and not to her taste.

At first she refuses to be showered, then accepts a shower and says it was a good experience, then demurs a few days later, maintaining that an assistant poured water over her head.

The odour in the apartment briefly improves, then grows stronger. Home care reports that in the space of two weeks Mom has rejected a shower ten times in a row.

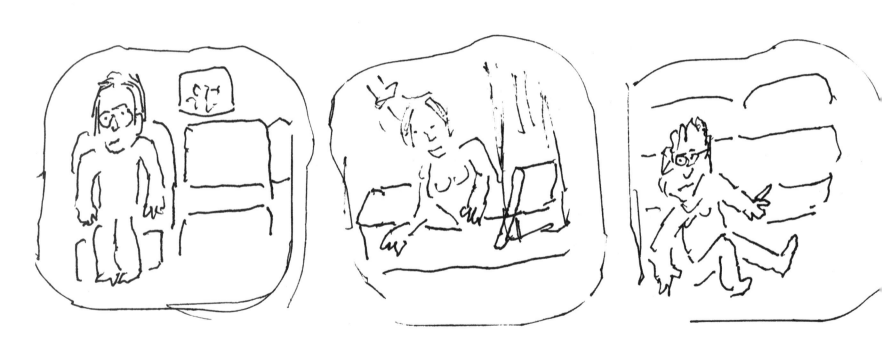

After a month of this, the pressure grows so overwhelming that entering my mother and brother's apartment is like touching down on the planet Jupiter. Crushed beneath the weight of tending my mother, Olivier sinks deep into the couch. He says little, but looks and sounds enormously depressed. My mother, accustomed to decades of running her life — doing her own laundry, straightening up the house, planning and cooking meals — struggles to carry on as before, and fails. Liv strives to pitch in, but when he offers to prepare a meal or do the wash he's hindered by his own inexperience and the fact that nothing ever meets Mom's standards. Mom rebuffs home care's offers of assistance as well so clothes don't get washed, counters don't get wiped, floors don't get swept, groceries don't get purchased, meals go uncooked. The plumbing inexplicably clogs and overflows repeatedly, leading me to believe she has been flushing her Depend undergarments down the toilet, despite having a special bin provided for them. Of course, if Mom's not eating right, neither is Olivier. Nic and I bring meals over, and perform quick cleanups, but the situation becomes so chaotic that Olivier flees to his social programs as early as he can each morning. At the same time he's deeply torn because of the powerful sense of loyalty he feels for my mother.

From Mom's perspective, however long Olivier is gone is too long. She's lonely. She's confused. She frets about what may have happened to him each time he leaves, and while I'm at work she routinely calls Cheryl to ask if she knows where he is. When Liv warns my mother that he'll return late, she forgets and panics — but regardless of when he returns, nothing makes her happy. She can't hear him speak and complains that he mumbles. She expects him to anticipate when she's thirsty, and is irritated when he doesn't. Her arthritis aches, her hip replacements grind, she contracts an ugly-looking leg infection. She's in pain, and frustrated each time she rises to get a drink or go to the washroom. She can't sleep. She's suspicious of everyone. Each home care intervention — designed to make her life more comfortable — ends in confrontation and commotion, which raises Olivier's anxiety further, prompting him to flee even faster.

They spend their nights watching television. By nine, my mother rises with a groan, grasps her walker and, shoving it ahead of her, retires to her bedroom. My brother swallows his medication, channel surfs, extinguishes the lights, and collapses into an unmade bed.

My mother's falls become a regular occurrence. One night her legs give out as she is making her way to the washroom and she decides, rather than to call for help, to spend eight hours on the floor waiting for Liv to wake.

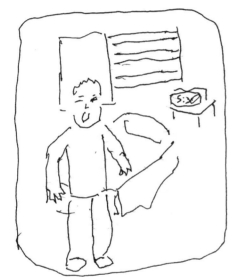

I AWOKE AT 5:30.

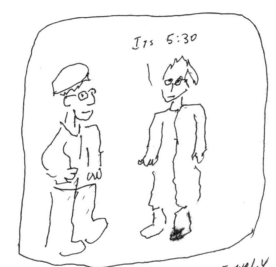

Its 5:30

MOM SAID I WAS TOO EARLY FOR THE BUS. I WAS JUST TRYING GET THE 6:00 BUS

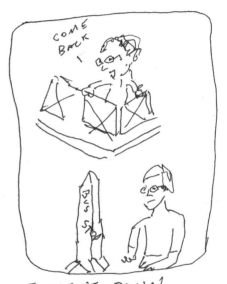

COME BACK

I WENT DOWN TO THE BUS STOP. I THOUGHT I HEARD MOM, BUT JUST WANTED TO GO.

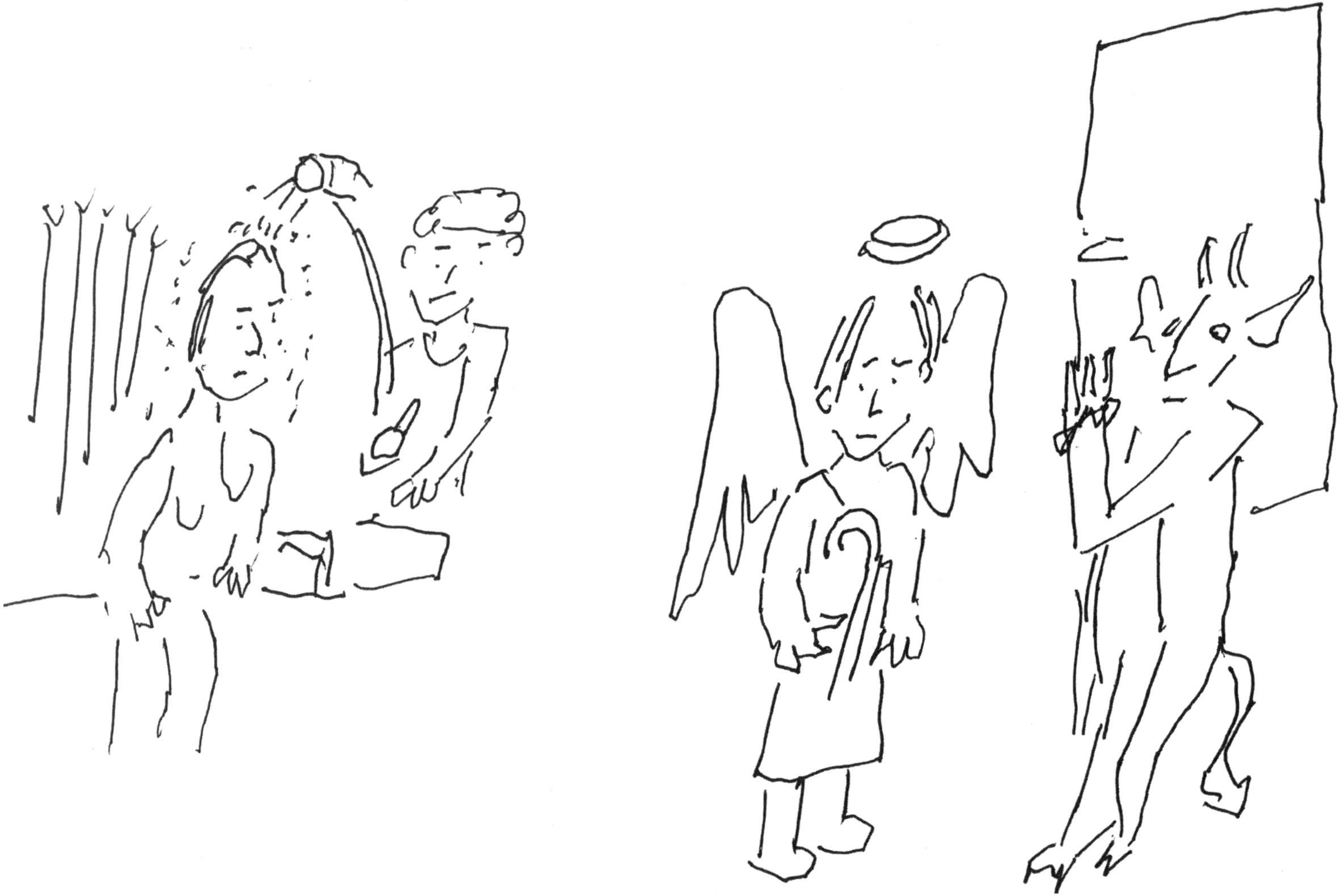

It becomes increasingly clear that Mom's refusal to accept help and her insistence that she decline in her own home, in her own time and on her own terms, is accelerating her deterioration and dragging Olivier down with her.

Nic, Liv, and I convene a meeting. We pull two chairs in from the dining room, Liv takes his place on the sofa, and Mom sits in her usual high-backed wooden chair. I outline the situation for my mother. Her hygiene and health are worsening and the apartment has fallen into disrepair. No matter how she dislikes it, she needs someone to come in, clean up, and prepare meals. Her legs have become swollen and infected. She needs someone to administer her medication and to give her showers.

When my mother denies all these facts, I bluntly point out that the apartment smells, and that she smells, whereupon she launches into an involved explanation of how the sponge bath is an art she perfected during the war which, when skillfully applied, provides a complete and thorough cleaning.

Nic interrupts to ask how, given that she has trouble reaching the coffee cup on the side table next to her, she imagines she would have the dexterity or balance to administer a complete sponge bath? And as evidence of her failure, he says, there's the smell. She has to accept home care's help.

"Help," she interrupts. "They are the *opposite* of helpful!" She complains that the home care employees are too young — mere teenagers. They are too dim — they don't know how to sweep or boil water or make a bed. They create more problems than they fix.

The harder we press her, the more she digs in. The dispute turns heated and then unhinged. Mom makes wild claims about the assistants. They swear, she says. They steal. They deliberately plant things in her way to trip her. Frustrated at his inability to make Mom understand how desperate the situation is and how short of solutions we are, Nic's voice rises.

"These problems won't go away," he shouts. "Things are bad already. They'll get worse unless you accept help. What can we do?"

"Whatever," she snaps back, "whatever! Just kill me."

Two days later, I return to the apartment early in the morning to try once more. Liv has gone out to his peer support group. Mom is in her bedroom, perched on the edge of her bed. She waves for me to come and help, but it's difficult to understand what she needs because she hasn't slipped her dentures in. When I ask what the problem is, she tells me — at least, as far as I can understand — that she can't stand. I look about the room for her walker. Frankly, I don't know how she got into bed, because it's parked in the living room.

I fetch the walker and position it next to her. Where are her dentures, I ask? Missing, she replies as she grips the walker, and tries and fails to haul herself up. After two or three attempts, it's clear that she hasn't the strength to accomplish the task.

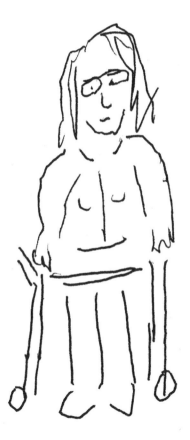

I'm hesitant to do a full lift, because this can result in her panicking, but I'm not sure what else to do, so I bend down, reach beneath her arms, and pull. She grabs the walker — doesn't say thank you, but doesn't scream either — and makes her way to the washroom.

While she's freshening up, I embark on a futile hunt for the dentures. I'm concerned that she may be unable to rise off the toilet — I've had to lift her off once before — but she returns from the washroom without incident. I offer her a Tim's breakfast sandwich and some coffee. While she gums on the English muffin I ask again where her dentures might have gone?

"Stolen," she says.

"Stolen?" I repeat. "By whom?"

"The plumber," she replies, and then goes on to claim that she'd dropped her dentures in a glass of water in the washroom. A plumber had come by to repair the toilet once more, and when he left, he pocketed them.

"What," I ask, "would a plumber possibly want with your old used dentures?"

My mother offers a tortured explanation which, boiled down to its essence, is that people stick it to the elderly. This is obviously a dead end.

"Let's think a moment. If you didn't put your dentures in a glass of water, where might you have placed them?"

She attempts to describe what I surmise is a white carrying case, but as is usual these days when she can't find the exact words she becomes agitated. "The white, the white, the white!" she exclaims, growing louder with each repetition, while at the same time making vaguely boxy gestures with her hands.

Not wanting to agitate her further, I abandon the interrogation and just assure her I'll make a more thorough search for them later.

Once she is calm and drinking her coffee, I seize the opportunity to promote the benefits of a supportive living facility. Rising in the morning has obviously become an impossible task. She loses things regularly. I remind her how often she has fallen, how many bruises she has accumulated as a result, how lonely she feels when we're all at work. The Bow Valley facility, for instance, is located in her old neighbourhood and would offer her companionship and the kind of care that she needs.

To my astonishment she nods and says that it sounds like a good idea. I suppress an enormous sigh of relief, and caution her that she'll have to sign some forms. And, I add, there could be a wait before a placement becomes available.

Best to get after it soon, she responds. Buoyed by her positive response, and feeling that we're making progress, I talk her through the process. A monthly fee will be debited from her account to pay for her residency, but between the government pension she receives and the additional government assisted-living subsidy she will be provided, she shouldn't have to dip into her savings. She listens and says that it sounds like it could work.

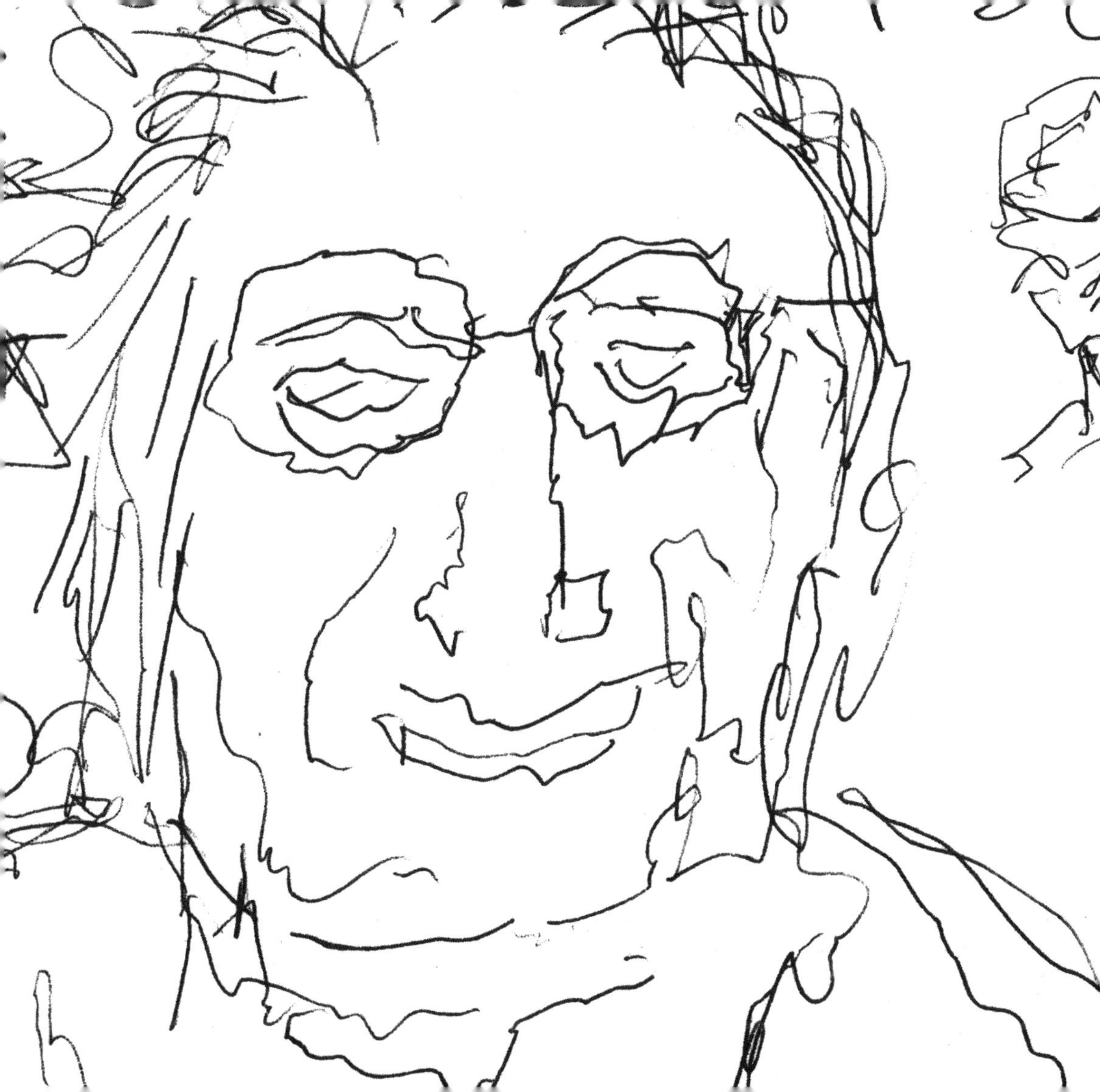

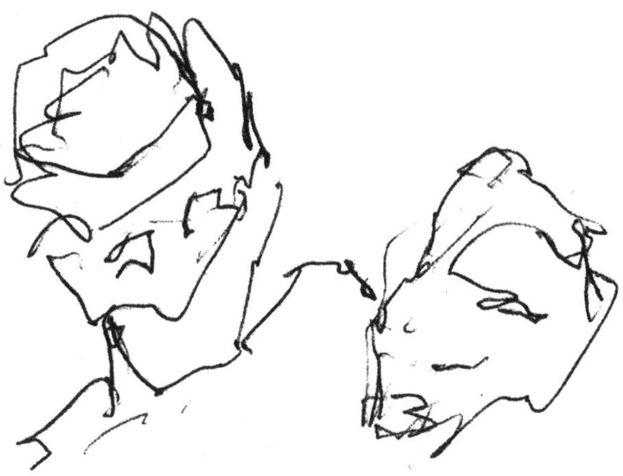

A huge weight lifts off of me. Then I realize that there are no witnesses. No one to attest to this milestone. I grab the notebook that we have been using to exchange weekly thoughts and stories, and write this moment up, including the details of our previous discussion. I read it back to her. She confirms everything!

At last, she seems to understand that the present living arrangement can't carry on, and that change is required.

She agrees!

Thank heavens!

The very next day she has forgotten our conversation entirely, and cares nothing for the paragraph I've scrawled in our write-and-respond book.

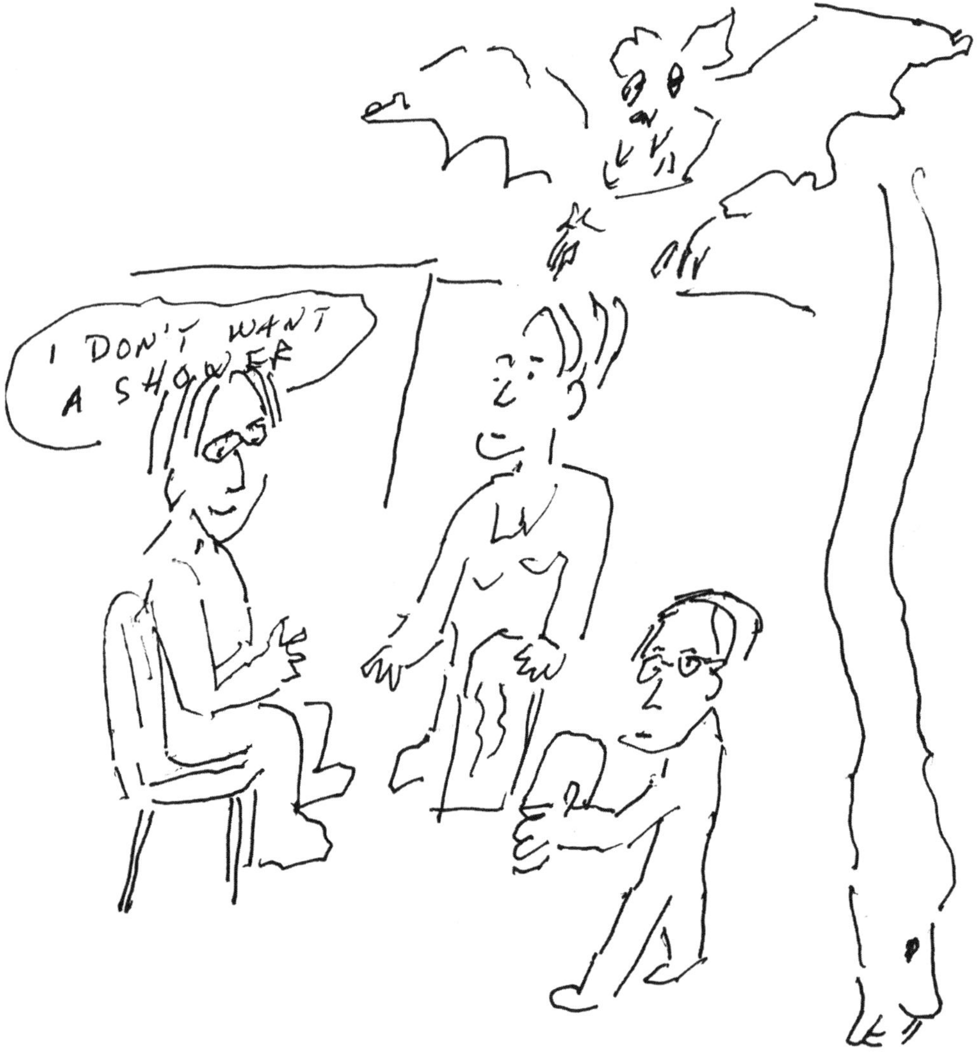
I DON'T WANT A SHOWER

Nevertheless, Nic calls home care to inquire where we are with pursuing placement at a supportive living facility.

"Nowhere," the supervisor informs him. "The previous entry was terminated."

Surprised, Nic asks why and is told that during one of the in-home visits, Mom stated she was no longer interested. Why weren't the rest of us advised, Nic inquires. She assumed we knew. If he wishes, she will re-enter the paperwork and mark it urgent.

Which means that we can expect to hear from the placement coordinator in four to eight weeks, and even after this individual determines the type of residence Mom should move to, we can expect to wait anywhere from six months to two years for a placement.

Two years. How can this situation possibly be sustained another two years?

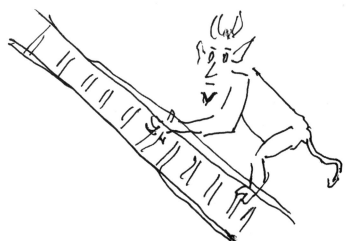

My mother spends her days perched on her chair surveying the world through her living room window, lonely, angry, ill, her only certainty being that she will not, absolutely will not, accept help.

Olivier tells me that one of his social workers has said she might have helpful advice, but when I call her, rather than offering advice, she launches into a loud lecture. Do I realize what a difficult situation Olivier is in? Do I understand what it's like for him living with my mother? I tell her I have an idea. Do I know how troubled my mother is? I tell her I have a pretty good notion of how troubled my mother is. She warns me that Olivier is anxious and depressed, the situation isn't healthy, and I have to do something. I tell her we're trying. I tell her it's complicated. I thank her. I hang up.

What I want to say is, "Thank you so much for stating the obvious but what exactly do you suggest?" I want to say, "My mother and brother are co-owners of an apartment that they presently cannot sell, nor do they have an interest in moving out separately. They're both fragile in their own way. If you have a solution, *give it to me*. I am totally in the market for solutions."

We take Mom to the seniors' health centre at the Rockyview Hospital to have her hips examined and to get some fall prevention strategies. The clinic will also provide an assessment of her general health.

I schedule an extra hour to prepare her for the appointment, and wish I'd planned for three. Everything requires more time and effort than I'd anticipated. Dressing takes time — she doesn't want my help, but teeters on the verge of falling each time she slips an arm through a sleeve. Breakfast takes time. Making sure she has everything takes time — including the purse she insists on slinging over her shoulder whenever she goes out and which is so heavy it throws her off balance. Walking to the car, getting into the car, finding and securing the seat belt, getting out of the car.

We arrive late. Nic is waiting with a wheelchair at the clinic entrance and he and I accompany our mother into the examining room. Two women rise from their seats to greet us: one short and youngish, the doctor, and one older and taller, the physiotherapist.

My mother is polite, but guarded. Her hearing impairment again presents an obstacle, so the doctor and physiotherapist adjust their seats and face her directly. The doctor asks a few general questions, which my mother fields pretty well, explaining that she has arthritis, a leg injury she received in the war, a couple of hip replacements which are now deteriorating, and that a brain aneurism she experienced in the nineties left her with some residual dizziness. The doctor probes a little further about the aneurism. At first Mom responds coherently, but then she jumps tracks and recounts her flight from the Russians following World War II. The aneurism was bad, she concludes, but nothing compared to the trials of the war. The doctor and physiotherapist wait patiently as the story draws to a close, then test her memory and cognition. Following that, she is persuaded to go down the hall with the physiotherapist to test her range of motion and stability.

Once she has left the room, the doctor gazes across the table at Nic and me and says, "She's in pretty bad shape, hey?"

We agree.

"Have you spoken with her about applying for help at home?" she asks.

We share what we've done so far, and our lack of success. She nods sympathetically, makes a few notes, then asks, "Have you considered assisted living?" We tell her that we placed her name on a list, she cancelled it, and now we've put her name back on it.

"What would she like to do?" the doctor asks.

"Die of natural causes in her apartment," I tell her.

The doctor grimaces. I assume she hears that a lot. She diagnoses Mom as suffering from some dementia, but feels she may be able to remain at home if there are sufficient supports in place. She adds a caution that this kind of medical situation can evolve quickly, so she'd like to see Mom return in a few months for a follow-up.

She writes up her appraisal and provides my mother with a copy. Mom didn't care for the appointment, doesn't like the assessment, and as we drive home, loudly expresses her suspicion that the woman we saw wasn't a doctor at all.

Thanksgiving approaches. Nic's family have gone out of town and Cheryl's sister has invited Cher and me and our kids to her lakeside cabin. We try to figure out how Mom might make it to the gathering, but there are stairs at the cabin, which present a problem, and lately she has become so troubled by sudden sounds and so emotionally volatile that it makes participation in larger get-togethers almost impossible. And there's her refusal to shower. I urge Cher to go on ahead, and tell her I'll try to join her and our daughters later.

Rather than allowing the day to pass unacknowledged for Liv and Mom, I invite them out for a picnic. I pick them up in the early afternoon and, together, Liv and I help Mom into the car. I purchase some chicken, salad, and fries, and we head out to Glenbow Ranch Provincial Park.

This park, only fifteen minutes northwest of their apartment, is situated on a crest overlooking the river valley and mountains. Wooden picnic tables dot the ridge just a short hike from the parking lot.

I lift the walker from the trunk, carry it to the passenger side, and help Mom out of the car. She slowly straightens, grasps the walker, then shoves it ahead in the aggressive inchworm style she's adopted. A paved path exits the fenced parking lot and winds out along a grassy meadow. We veer from the path briefly and make our way through short grass prairie to one of the picnic tables. The thick scent of sage and willow rises and fills the air.

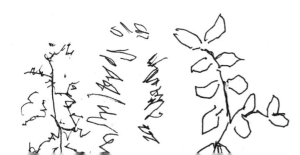

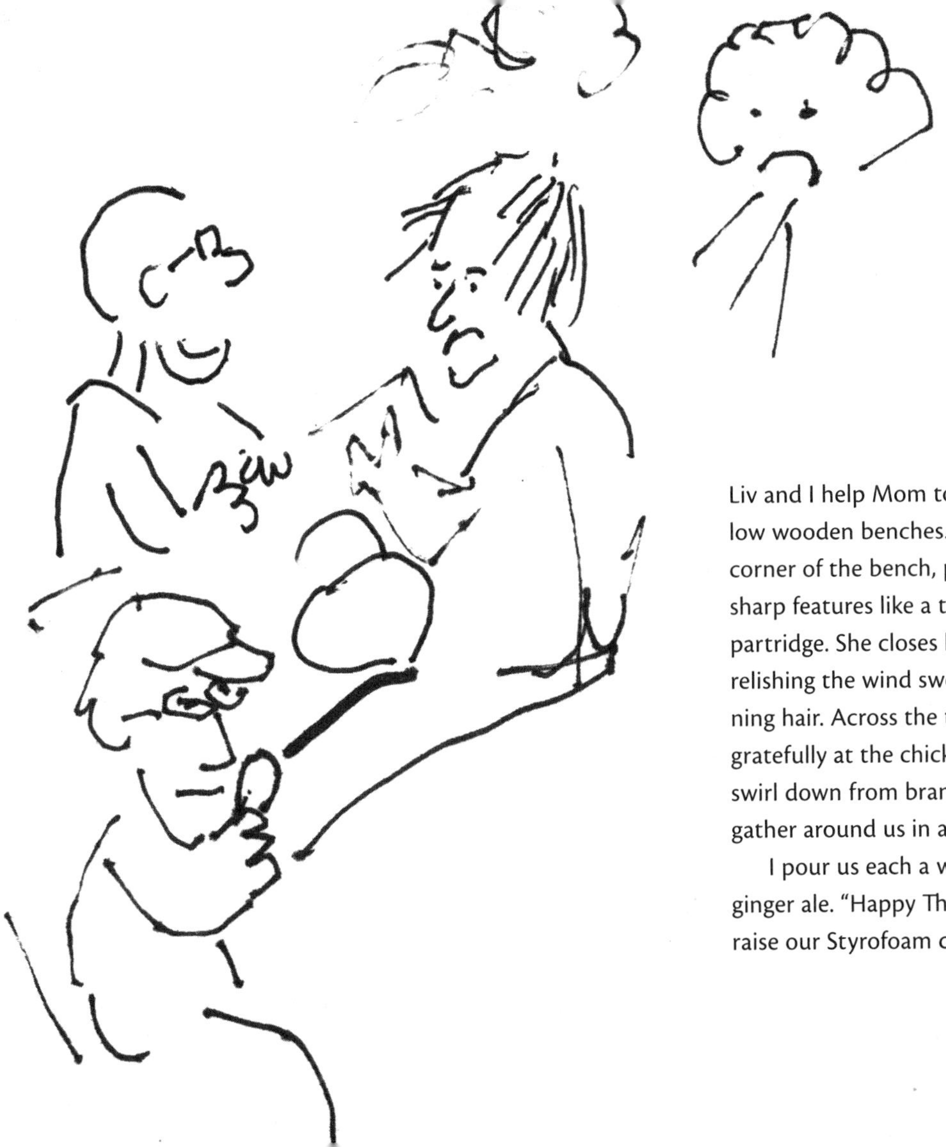

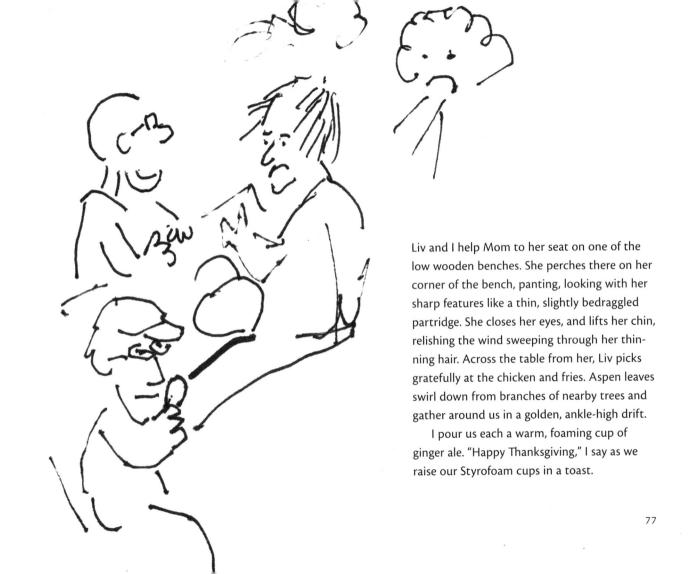

Liv and I help Mom to her seat on one of the low wooden benches. She perches there on her corner of the bench, panting, looking with her sharp features like a thin, slightly bedraggled partridge. She closes her eyes, and lifts her chin, relishing the wind sweeping through her thinning hair. Across the table from her, Liv picks gratefully at the chicken and fries. Aspen leaves swirl down from branches of nearby trees and gather around us in a golden, ankle-high drift.

I pour us each a warm, foaming cup of ginger ale. “Happy Thanksgiving,” I say as we raise our Styrofoam cups in a toast.

HOW MUCH
TIME DO I HAVE

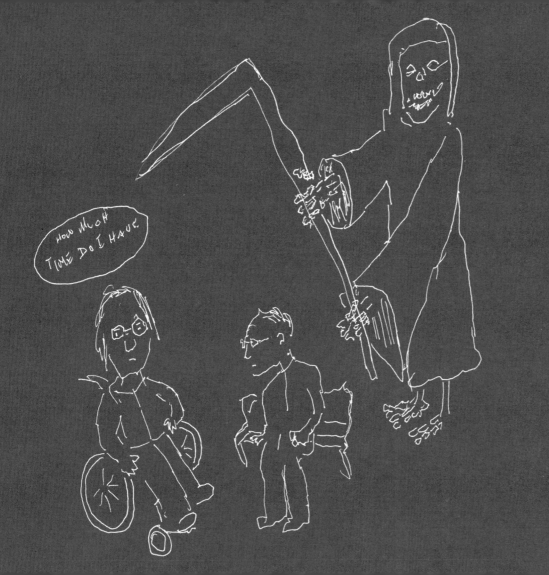

I dream about Liv. He's struggling to complete a difficult project. He has to drive to Edmonton to paint a house — when did he start a house-painting business? — and will return later that same evening. I find that worrying. It's a two-and-a-half-hour drive to Edmonton, and it will be dark when he returns. He hates driving, and his car is ancient and unreliable. Plus he'll be tired. What if he falls asleep at the wheel? What if the car fails?

I wake up, realize it's only a dream, but can't shake the compulsion to call him. It's early, but as it turns out not early enough: he's already left. Instead I get my mother who is happy to talk, but confused about why I've phoned. I chat for a few moments, tell her I'll visit later in the day, and hang up. I try reaching Liv on his cell but don't get an answer. He only turns it on to call out.

Slowly rubbing the receiver against my forehead, I fret and watch rain streak the living room window. I think about my brother and mother, confined in their decaying apartment, about how often Mom has been telling Liv — telling us all — "I want to die in my apartment. Just let me die in my apartment." It's not a directive so much as it is a prayer.

Just let me die in my apartment. If only it were that easy. If only, when things got too desperate Death could be summoned like a repairperson or pizza delivery. If only when you were weary of life, or are no longer able to cope, you could simply invoke Death, who would appear like the hero of a bad novel to draw things to a graceful conclusion. But the truth is, Death is incompetent. Summon all you wish, he never arrives according to schedule.

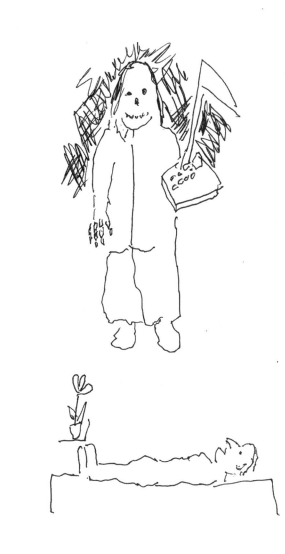

NO! NO! NO!

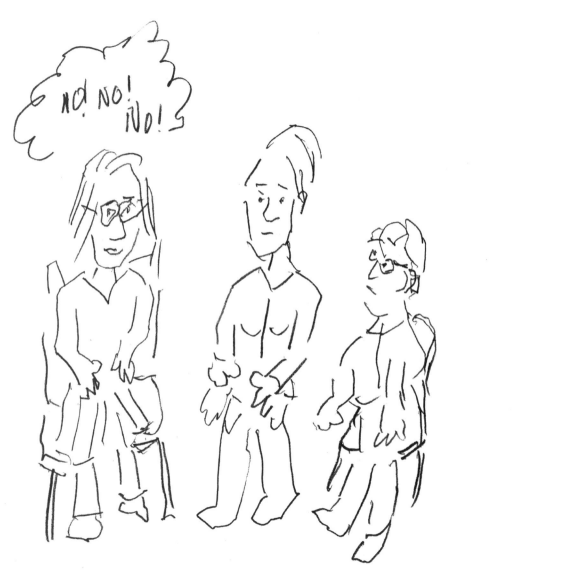

NO NO! NO!

The following week is a train wreck. Nic phones to tell me that he received a call at work from home care asking him to come to the apartment. Mom had fallen but wouldn't permit the home care assistant to touch her. When Nic arrived from work, she had been on the floor three hours. After helping her up, he wanted to offer her something to eat but the fridge was empty.

Two days later Nic calls when I'm in the middle of teaching a graduate class. Mom has fallen once more and won't allow her home care worker to help. Nic is across town and in the middle of meetings and can't get there. Luckily, I'm able to terminate the class and drive over.

She's on the floor of the living room, propped against the couch. The worker has fled the building. I bite my lip in frustration, lift Mom to her chair, and ask *why* she wouldn't let the home care worker assist her — that's what they're there for. She just shakes her head.

Home care notifies us that they will no longer send workers, as Mom has refused all assistance for an extended period.

The next day, the chair of the condominium board calls to inform us that there have been numerous complaints about the odour and the troubled comings and goings at Mom and Liv's apartment. When she followed up with a visit she found the conditions unacceptable. She points out that the condominium board has the right to terminate a contract if they feel the condominium isn't being properly maintained.

Nic, Liv, and I convene another early Sunday morning meeting. Mom can detect something in the wind and sits ramrod straight in her chair, her eyes darting from one of us to the other. I start by letting her know that the head of the condominium board has called to insist that we take action, that the board has the right to expel a client who isn't maintaining their property.

Rather than acknowledging the chaotic living conditions, my mother alleges that she is the victim of an elaborate conspiracy perpetrated by the condominium board, home care, "the doctors," and maybe the entire health care system.

None of these parties have an interest in seeing her move, I object; they would much rather she stayed in her apartment, if she could maintain it, but she can't. The phone call from the chair of the condominium board is just another sign that she needs help.

The word *help* triggers an instant furious outpouring. In a refrain that has become all too familiar, she now claims that the "help" is worse than useless. It's malign. Unskilled workers invade her home and treat it like a dump. They send men instead of women to clean her. They toss garbage into the sink and block the plumbing. They steal from her, then deny it. They're rough, they're rude. They shout at her. They hold her head under the water when they shower her. She wants none of it.

How would she know if the help works, I demand. She never lets them do anything. She won't let them clean the house or do the laundry, won't let them shower her, won't let them make the bed, won't let them pick her up when she falls, won't even let them sweep. If they're useless, I tell her, it's because she won't let them be of use.

They don't send qualified staff, my mother snaps. They send criminals or babies.

Nic interrupts to tell Mom that no one is stealing from her — her dentures, which she claimed were stolen, were later found wedged under her mattress. No one is persecuting her. The head of the condominium board has no connection to home care. The situation in the apartment simply isn't sustainable anymore. Something has to be done. It's time for her to move into an assisted living facility.

My mother glares. "Kill me," she says. "Just kill me."

"That's not an option," Nic replies evenly.

"If the condominium board orders you out," I ask, "where will you go? Where will Liv go?"

"We need to get more help for you," Nic continues, "and the only solution we can see is for you to move into assisted living."

"We have to do something, Mom," Liv interjects quietly.

"Whatever," she repeats, but I can see that she is caught off guard by Olivier's participation in what she sees as our collective betrayal.

"But do you understand?" Nic presses.

An uncomfortable silence follows as Mom blinks away tears, then turns away, angry, hurt, and humiliated. "Fine," she says, staring out the window. "Whatever."

Which is as close to agreement as we ever come.

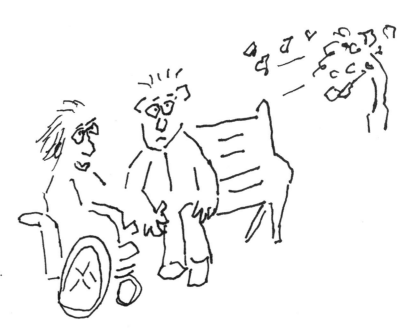

When I call the seniors' health centre to learn how we can accelerate the move to assisted living, I'm told we will need another assessment to determine her level of incapacity.

"Is that absolutely necessary?" I ask. "She won't want another assessment. She won't submit to another assessment."

The doctor is understanding; apparently this kind of resistance is common. "Try to convince her, but if you can't, you may have to lie to her."

I hang the phone up. Lie to her. Perfect.

As it turns out, though, I don't have to lie. My mother's infected, swollen leg worsens, and gives her so much pain that she is eager to see someone.

The day of the appointment I arrive in the early morning and find my mother more tired than usual. I help her up, steady her as she grasps the walker, walk alongside her to the washroom. She's in there a long time and I weigh whether I should call to her, but she suddenly pops out, shoving her walker ahead of her to her chair. There's the standard anxious moment as she determines how she'll descend/fall from standing to sitting.

Once seated, she groans and complains that she had a terrible night because a noisy party kept her awake. I'm surprised. The majority of residents in the complex are elderly and I can't imagine anyone hosting an event so raucous that others would be disturbed.

"Party?" I ask. "Were the next-door neighbours loud?"

"No," she says, gesturing to the living room, "here in the condominium. Olivier had people over·drinking until all hours."

Nothing could be more absurd than the idea of Olivier hosting some kind of midnight raver, but she paints a picture as detailed as it is farfetched. When I press her on inconsistencies, she simply insists that she saw what she saw.

"How did you get out of bed to observe these partiers?" I ask. "I had to help you up today. You can't view the living room from your bed."

My mother pauses and frowns. "Oh no!" she fumes. "I didn't see it. I can't have seen it! I'm demented! I'm *demented!*"

My heart sinks, not because I haven't encountered delusions before, but because I have.

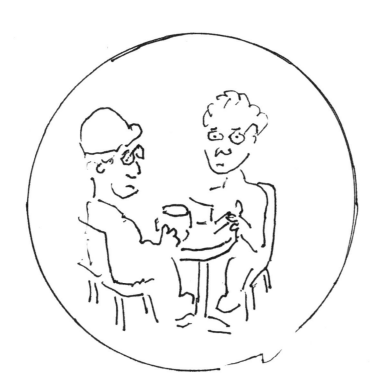

In the throes of their psychotic episodes, both Ben and Olivier experienced elaborate hallucinations and delusions. But living alongside someone in a delusional or psychotic state is more challenging than most people realize. You are constantly strategizing for events that defy strategy. Things that you think should work, won't. Things that you think should please, don't. Offers of help are viewed as threats. Real dangers are ignored and fanciful dangers take on a terrifying dimension. Psychosis causes such a fracture in any kind of shared reality that it's difficult to carry out the simplest activity. You end up improvising each day, because any regular, planned for, traditional exchanges won't work. It's exhausting and I dread dealing with it once more.

I shelve our discussion of drunken revelry and shepherd my mother out the door, and we drive to the Rockyview Hospital in uncomfortable silence. For my mother, travel is now a considerable hardship — and she is suspicious of what my brothers and I are trying to do, regardless of how we frame it. I don't know what will happen when we arrive. It's possible that she will simply curse the doctors out. She may refuse to leave the car at all. I try to find ways to discuss the situation that she won't find upsetting, but her mental instability has rendered every conversation perilous.

Dementia is often described as a kind of "decline" — as though it were a leisurely descent down a gently rolling hillside. Nothing could be farther from the truth. Dementia isn't a decline: it's a plummet from a precipice. And as you fall you strike against the rocky cliff face, each strike removing another portion of who you were. Strike! — there goes your short-term memory. Strike! — there goes your ability to read. Strike! — there goes your recognition of faces.

Once again, Nic has a wheelchair ready at curbside when we arrive. We proceed to the seniors' health centre, and Mom has her leg examined. She's provided with a prescription for the infection, as well as for a bladder infection that's gone undiagnosed. Even though the pills will be placed in a blister pack providing the precise dosage for each day of the month, she'll need assistance taking them — the last time she received a blister pack she went through a week of pills in a morning. The doctor asks how Mom has been enjoying home care. My mother instantly launches into a tirade about their terrible ineptitude, then segues into a celebration of sponge bathing and concludes triumphantly that the rigours of her escape from Germany left her capable of facing all eventualities. The doctor nods. She tests my mother's memory. I'm shocked at how poorly she performs in comparison with her examination two months ago.

When Mom teeters out the door to have her mobility re-examined, the doctor tells Nic and me that our mother's physical health is seriously compromised and her mental capacity has diminished so significantly that she no longer has the ability to make sound judgments.

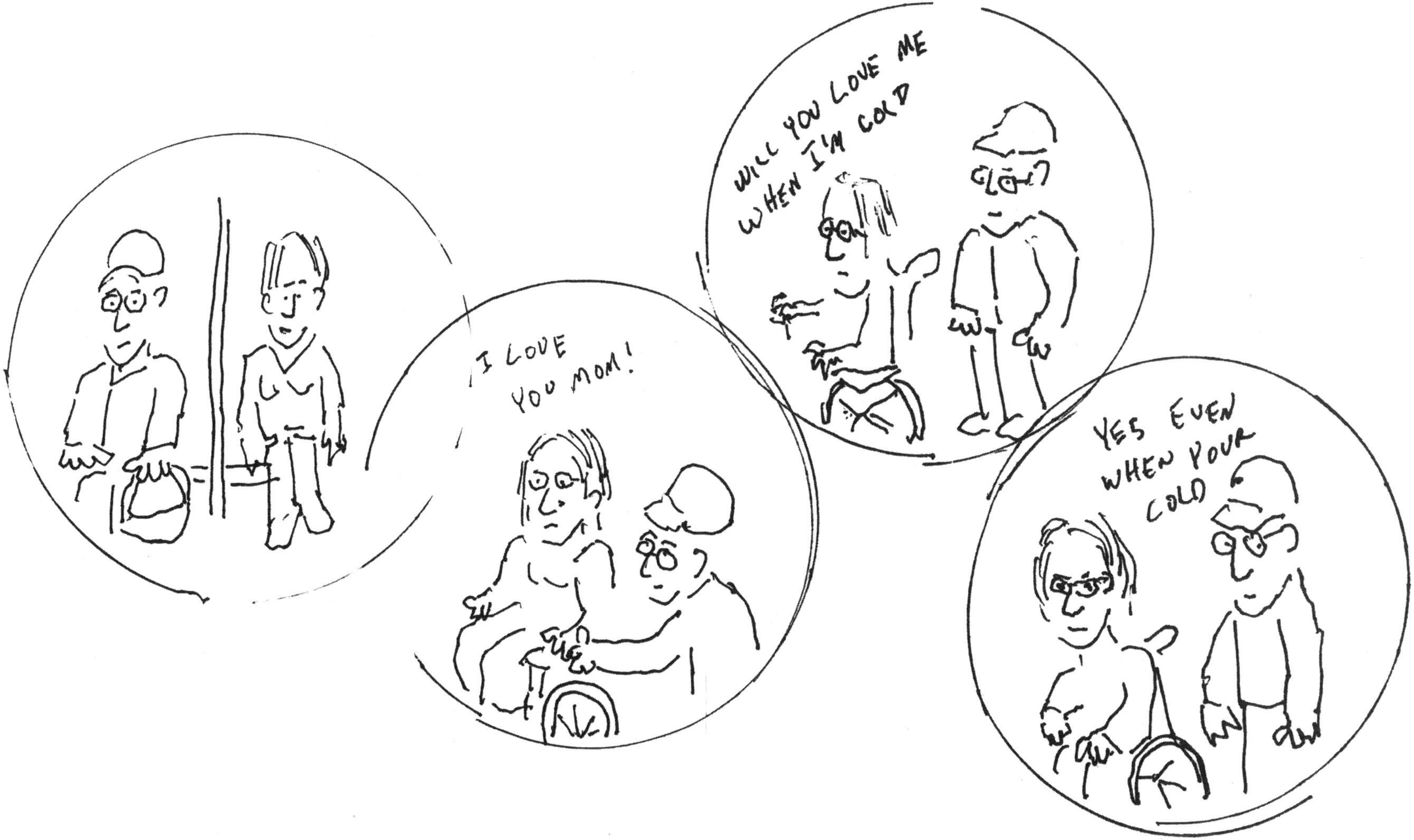
I LOVE YOU MOM!
WILL YOU LOVE ME WHEN I'M COLD
YES EVEN WHEN YOUR COLD

It's time to transition, the doctor tells us, and by "transition," she means it's time for my mother to abandon her home and the life she's lived. A room will be prepared for her in the transition unit of the Rockyview Hospital within a couple of weeks.

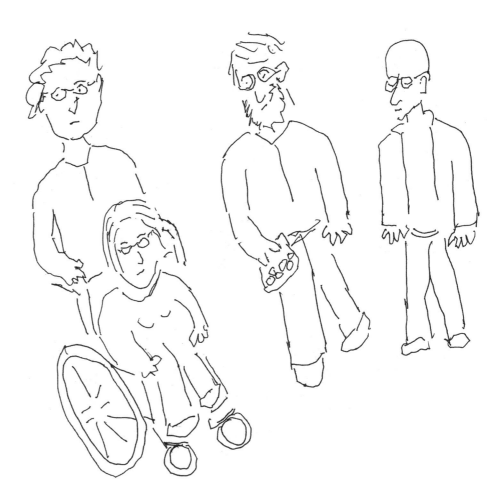

Two days later Nic calls to say that the Rocky-view emergency has processed the doctor's recommendation, so we can make the transfer earlier — say the weekend or even tomorrow. The emergency doctor on call will fill in the Form 1 assessment of incapacity and enter Mom into the hospital.

So, now, not a couple of weeks, but this weekend.

I TAKE THE
NUMBER 20

I MADE A WATER
COLOUR PAPER
STRETCH

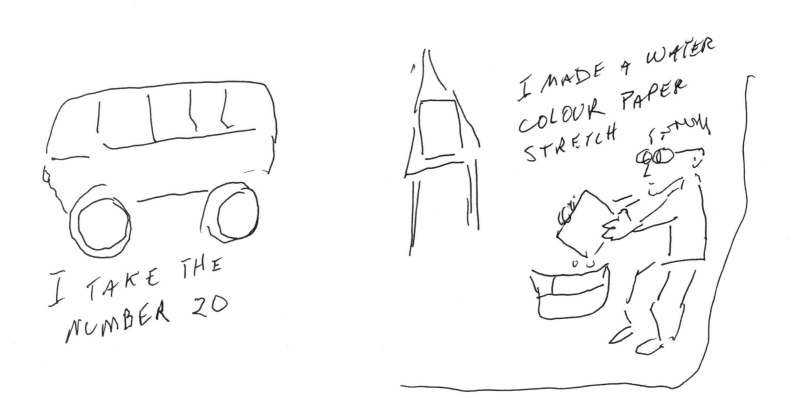

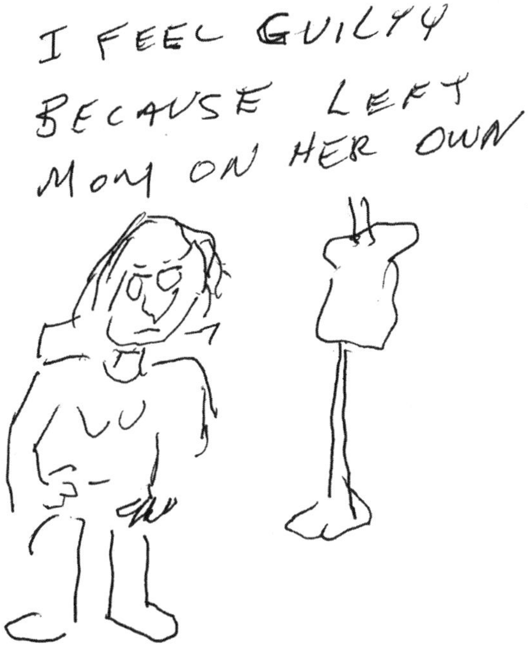
I FEEL GUILTY
BECAUSE LEFT
MOM ON HER OWN

Olivier and I meet for breakfast at the local Denny's, and over coffee I tell him we'll be taking Mom to the hospital on Friday morning. After she leaves the apartment, she won't return, so he'll be on his own until we sort things out.

He sighs heavily, turns to the window and studies the uninspiring, cigarette-strewn Denny's parking lot. He's silent a long, long time. Finally, I ask if he's going to be all right.

He nods, then sighs again. He says he guesses it means he has failed to take care of Mom.

That takes me by surprise. I assure him it's not his fault, nobody thinks it's his fault, and certainly it's not about his failure. I don't think it's about anybody's failure. It's about all of us trying to find some way to care for Mom. That's all.

"Is there anything you'd like us to do, to make things better for you?" I ask. "Do you want to move out or get a roommate?"

He shakes his head.

"Are you going to be okay?" I ask again.

He says he supposes he will, but looks anything but.

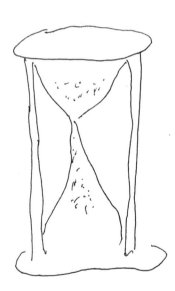

The day approaches and I'm sick with anxiety.

I go to the Y and run the track, past the treadmills, the elliptical machines, past the seniors leaning on the railing chatting, past the balance balls and the chin-up beams.

I try to think things through. I try to find a way forward that offers some kind of positive outcome, some strategy that won't result in Olivier becoming ill once more or my mother feeling betrayed.

I can't see a good outcome. I focus on running. I focus on breathing. I wait for my brain to clear. One more lap.

Viewing my mother through the present filter of her incapacity, it's almost impossible to recollect just how capable she once was.

Yet I remember the pride I felt in her one day when I was seven and playing with Nic at a schoolyard. An older tough attacked Nic, and though the boy was nearly my mother's height, when he lunged at my brother she suddenly snagged him by his wrist, flipped him to the ground, and sent him on his way.

At a time when most women her age couldn't drive, when my father couldn't drive, when being a "woman driver" was considered a pejorative, she insisted on obtaining her driver's licence. She founded and operated her own kindergarten, helped establish the Calgary chapter of the Unitarian Church, ran for election on the local school board and won, then sat on the Calgary board for thirteen years. She advocated for greater representation of women in administrative roles in the school system, advocated on behalf of new immigrants, helped introduce and promote the first English as a Second Language programs in the Calgary school system, was instrumental in introducing kindergartens into the public school system. She was busy, she was socially adept, she made some profoundly good decisions. Many decades following her retirement as a trustee, I still encounter former employees of the Calgary public school system who tell me my mother mentored, assisted, and inspired them.

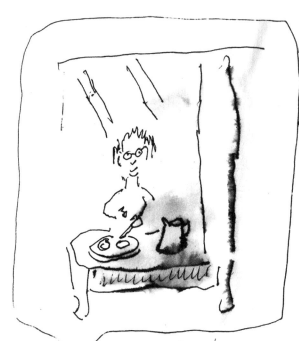

MY MOM ON SATURDAY WOULD GO TO BOW VALLEY AND COOK BREAKFAST FOR US KIDS

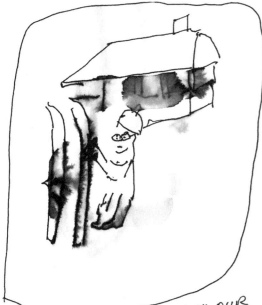

I AND BROTHERS WAX OUR SKIS AND CROSS COUNTRY

She was an inventive and resourceful parent. When she took us camping she wasn't like some of the other moms I knew, who waited in the car while their husbands set up the camp. She threw up the tent, chopped the wood, started the fire. Despite her war injury, she hiked with us up above the treeline into alpine meadows and was, I believe, happiest when surrounded by blooming columbines and mountain lilies.

We didn't have much money, but she managed to snag free tickets to the opera and took us to the Fledermaus. She enrolled us in ceramics classes, drove us downtown to participate in a weekly book club. In the winter she would wake us early, load up the car, cram us into the back seat, and speed out to a lake just north of the city. She stoked the cast iron stove of the cookhouse on the banks of the lake, and while breakfast cooked we'd lace up our skates and glide out onto the ice. Powerful winds swept that lake, but if you were able to withstand the shock of the cold air, you would unzip your jacket, feel it swell, and allow the wind to propel you over ice so clear you could count the pebbles of the rocky lakebed.

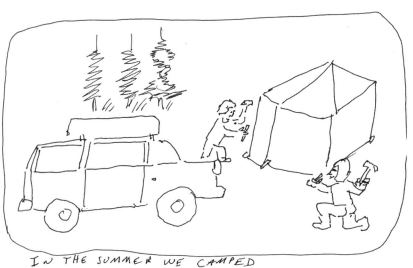

IN THE SUMMER WE CAMPED

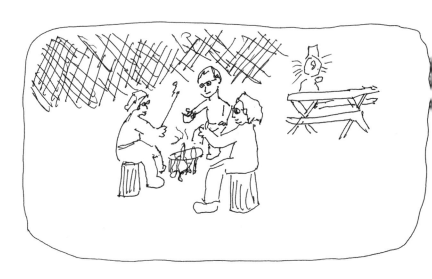

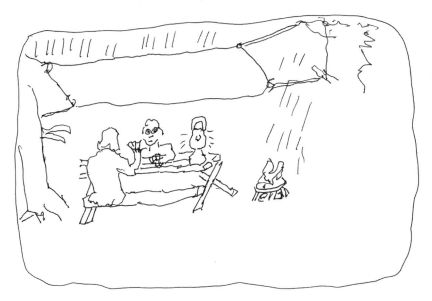

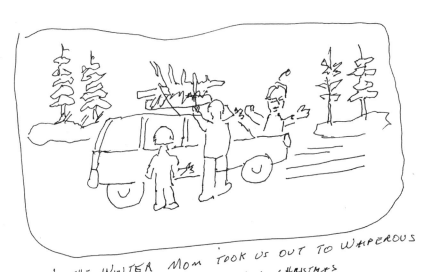

IN THE WINTER MOM TOOK US OUT TO WAIPEROUS
SO WE COULD CUT A TREE FOR CHRISTMAS

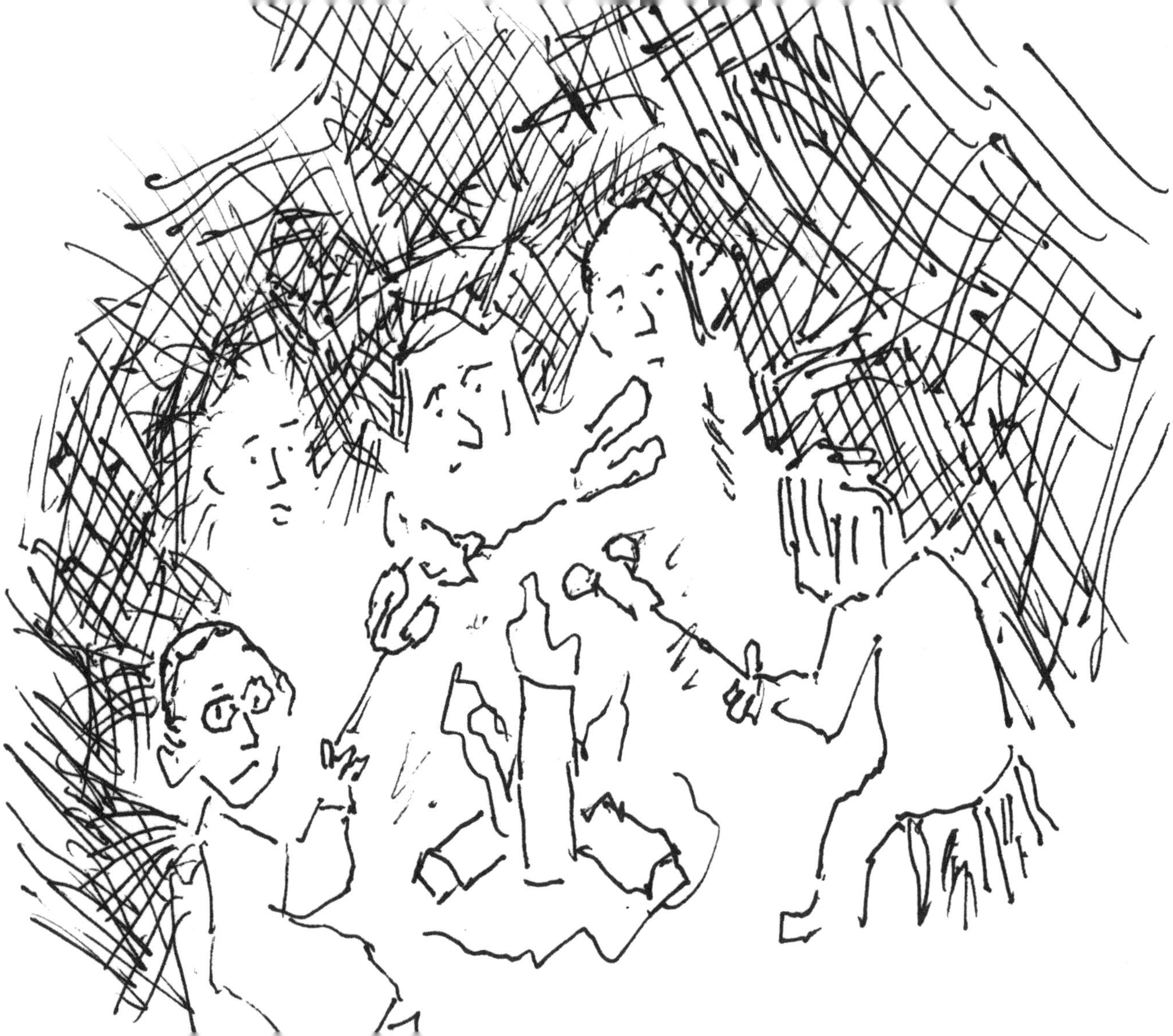

I don't know how to take her there.

It's two in the morning, I'm awake in my bed and every time I think about the impending journey – and it's impossible to stop thinking about it – I'm filled with dread.

I try to organize my thoughts. Nic and I have spoken with my mother about how "the transition" will proceed: that it will take time, that it will mean being checked into a hospital in the short term while the assessment is completed. Only after the assessment has been finalized will she be offered a placement at an assisted living facility. She's agreed.

But what does any of that mean, really? She agreed, yes – reluctantly – but will she remember the conversation later this morning when I arrive at the apartment? Will she remember it when we walk out the door? What if she refuses to go at the last minute? What if, at the hospital, she tells me she has changed her mind – if she turns about and pushes her walker out the hospital's main entrance?

I lie awake turning these things over. At three in the morning I rise and take my place at the dining room of my darkened home. I fire up the computer and make a list of the problems. There are dozens. I scroll down to a fresh page and begin a list of alternatives. There are none.

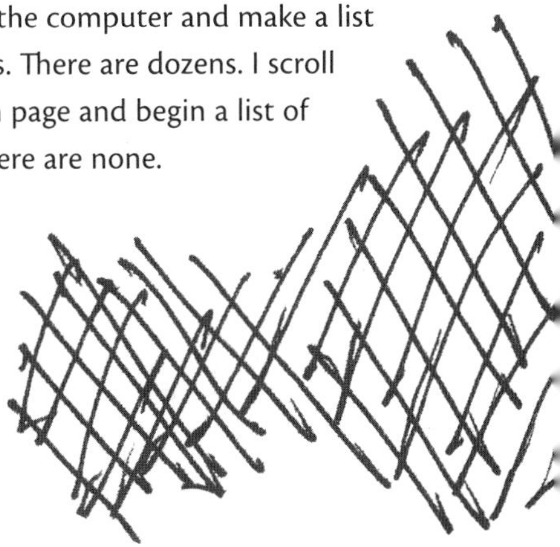

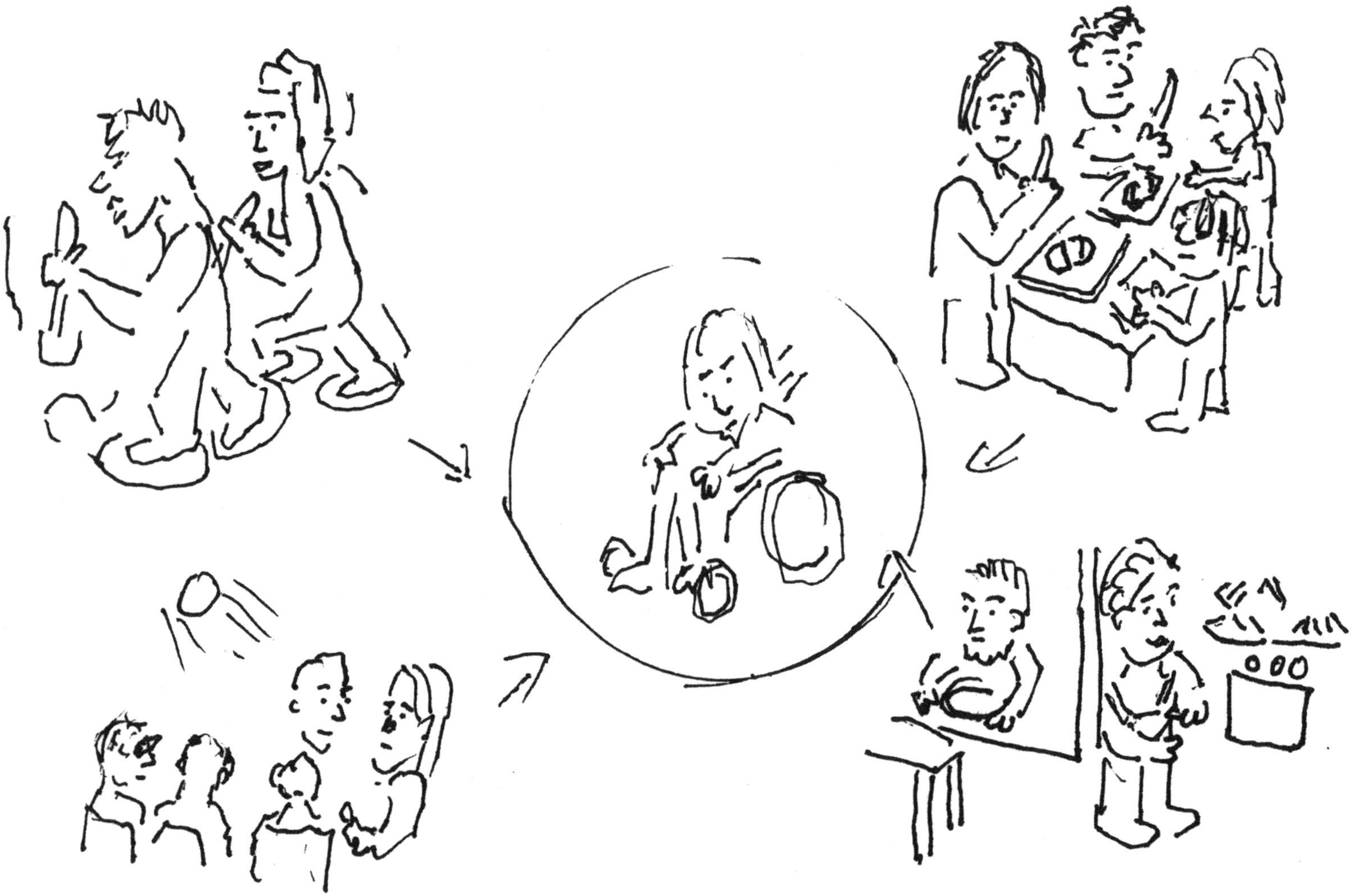

I arrive early. Liv has already left for the day. I help Mom rise from her bed. She lingers, dressing as I lay out our breakfast from Tim's. We eat, drink our coffee, and clean up, and then I say it's time to go. I ask if she has her health card. She nods, picks up her purse, loops its handle over her walker, and straightens her shoulders. I ask if she wants help with her purse. She says no, and reminds me that her whole life is in it. I open the apartment door. She locks it behind her, and I reflect that it's the last time she will do that.

Our descent in the elevator is silent, as is our slow march to the car. Once there, my mother negotiates the exchange from her walker to the passenger's seat, doing it, of course, without assistance. She feels about for level ground, then braces her ancient feet against the pavement. Slowly, she extends a skinny arm to find support, testing and rejecting first the headrest of the passenger seat, then the dusty upper ridge of the open car door, and eventually settling upon the arm rests of her walker. She turns, wavers, and performs a kind of awkward controlled fall into the car. I enter on the driver's side, buckle her in, and start the car.

It's February and frost clings to the branches of trees, dusting the roadways, transforming the landscape to a pale, ghostly grey. Spectral houses and shrubs and fences and lampposts flicker by with increasing speed as we turn onto the highway.

My mother relishes the ride, her eyes hungrily seizing on small details. As we cross town, she offers a disjointed commentary. How the city has changed over the years. How inappropriately for the temperature teenagers dress. She reminds me of all the summers we travelled by car together.

I recall those summers. It was an act of great bravery to ride with my mother. She was an anxious, uncomfortable, impulsive driver. Our journeys were conducted either well under the speed limit, as she hunched over the steering wheel, loudly lamenting the failings of fellow drivers, or kamikaze-like with her foot to the floor as she roared past the slower-moving logging trucks regardless of cars hurtling at us in the incoming lane.

Despite her driver's anxiety, she forced herself behind the wheel of a car each summer to escape the dust and heat, the poverty and bickering of our home. We ascended the eastern face of the Kicking Horse Pass, then descended west to the coast, our barely secured army surplus tent flapping from the car-rack like a flag. We traced snaky, winding, wet trucking roads, camped in thickets of Engelmann spruce and Douglas fir near mountain streams. My mother stretched our meager budget to impossible lengths by sending us to forage for berries, mushrooms, and herbs in the bushes near our campsites. She extended our menu, and made each foraging excursion seem like a treasure hunt.

When at last we arrived at the coast, we would erect our semi-permanent summer bivouac, and spend the remaining hot days swimming, digging for clams, reading paperback science fiction, and playing marathon games of rummy, crazy eights, and snap by lamplight throughout the night.

This was, without doubt, the best portion of my childhood. When I stretched out in in a sleeping bag, smelling cedar and listening to rain strike the tent, I felt alive. At the end of the day my mother would turn down the hissing Coleman lamp and tell my brothers and me to go to sleep. It was the last thing she said before the light winked out.

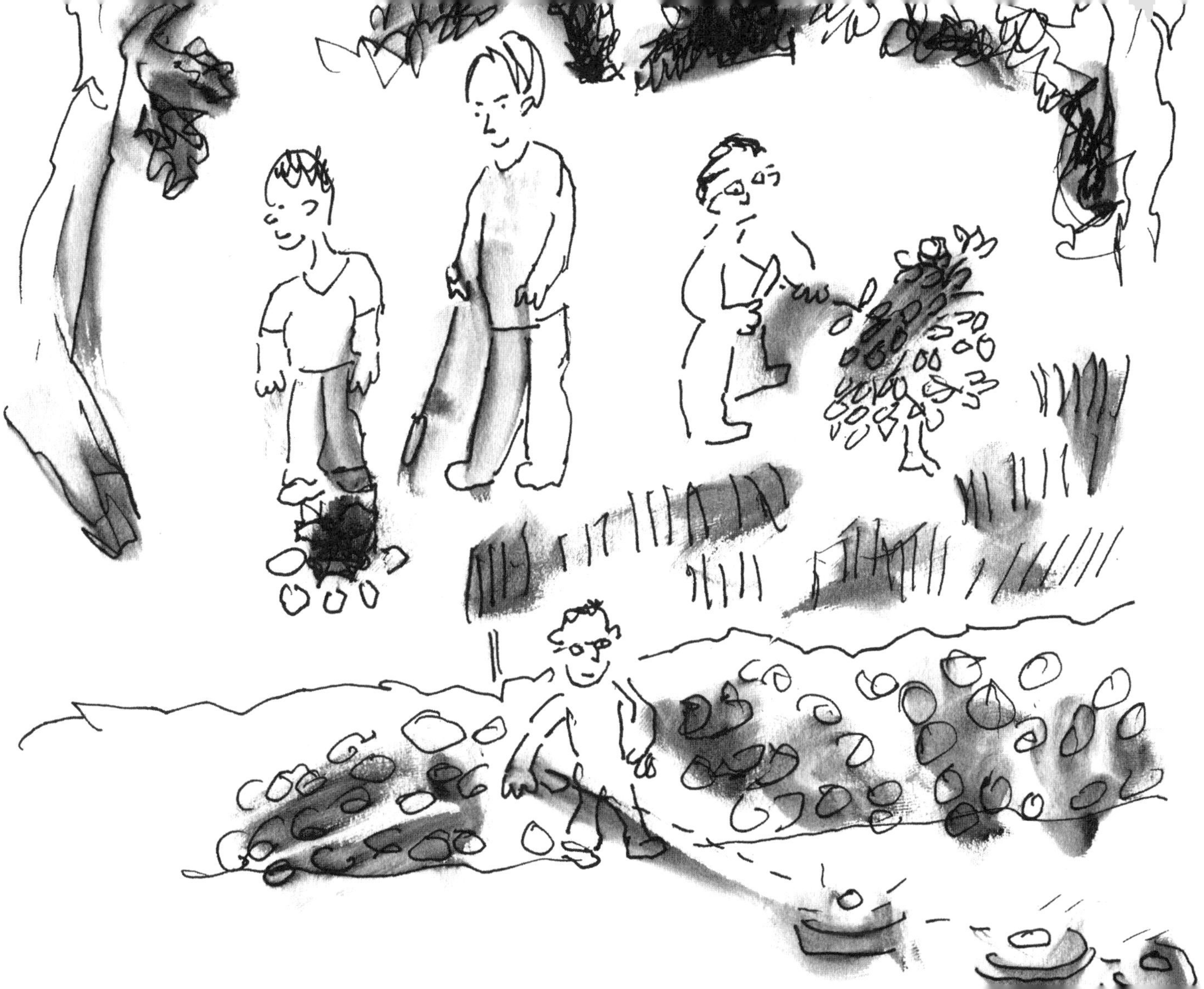

When we arrive at the hospital, I park, then walk to the entrance and borrow one of the hospital's wheelchairs. I return to the car and help Mom into it. We enter emergency, meet Nic, and take our place in line. Mom is registered, provided a green and white identification wristband. We park ourselves in the waiting room. Nic and I switch off, taking turns sitting with Mom, providing information, or fetching food and drink from the cafeteria. Restless, my mother demands to know what we are doing here? I explain again that it is part of the process of transition to a new facility. I remind her of the doctor's assessment and recommendations. She stops listening, and I'm uncertain how much she has actually absorbed.

Nevertheless, she appears calmer — and having visited hospitals on multiple occasions, she is familiar with the concept of waiting.

A nurse appears and takes Mom's blood pressure, then hands me a form requesting that I describe our mother's "lack of capacity." I fill it out. Eventually we are summoned and conducted through the locked doors of the emergency unit. The doors click shut behind us. Mom is wheeled into a tiny tent-like cubicle, framed by four grey, hanging curtains. Another nurse draws the front curtain closed and asks Mom to don a hospital gown. She refuses, and a team of two nurses swiftly convenes to facilitate the procedure. She is filthy, having refused a shower for months. The nurses don masks,

smocks, and gloves, and remain polite but determined as they descend on her. In a brief time she is changed and clean. When they are finished, she reclines on a cot, garbed in one of those inelegant open-backed gowns, and waits. One nurse lingers to gently comb my mother's fine hair and pin it back, and in so doing manages to restore some of my mother's dignity. It is a generous and completely unexpected gesture of grace.

Evening comes, and a nurse arrives to drop off a sandwich wrapped in plastic and coffee. Time drags. In the vestibule to our right a man vomits into a bucket, groans, and erupts again. An alarm is mysteriously triggered and just as mysteriously quelled. The night staff argue in low tones about rotation policy.

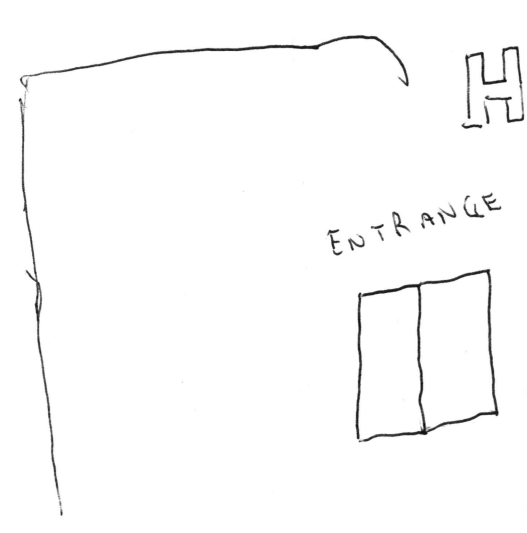

Another nurse arrives to take blood. She searches and probes, but, unable to find a vein until the third try, leaves a dark, grapefruit-sized bruise staining the inside of my mother's elbow. The resident doctor joins us, asks our mother a series of questions, records her answers that aren't really answers, signs the forms affirming her mental incapacity, and admits her to the hospital.

Another eight hours pass as we wait for a bed to become vacant, during which time Nic and I continue to spell each other off, either sitting with Mom or catching a nap. Mom sighs, grumbles to herself, then abruptly turns and demands to know why she is spending the night. When I remind her that she is here for tests to determine the level of care she'll require, her face hardens and she informs me she doesn't want or need tests. She wants to leave. I say that's not possible.

And suddenly she understands. I see it. I actually *see* the realization hit her, the understanding that she will never return home, and it strikes so suddenly and with such force that she recoils, and in order to maintain her composure and suppress her panic, she focuses on her sandwich. She carefully unwraps and then refolds the cellophane, stroking it smooth into a tidy, slick, compact square. She methodically consumes her meal, mouthful by slow mouthful, but when the last crumb disappears and there is no more to eat, nothing left to defer her crisis, it overwhelms her. Her body sags, her face crumples, she opens her mouth and sobs.

Nic and I exchange frozen glances. I don't know what to say. I haven't known what to say for weeks.

"Mom," Nic says softly, "it's going to be all right."

I hold her. "It isn't a punishment, Mom," I tell her. "We're only trying to find a way to keep you safe. We don't know how to cope any more when you fall, or when you refuse home care assistance. We have to be honest. We love you, but nothing else has worked. We need to try something new."

"Who," she sobs from behind her hands, "will take care of Olivier? Who will remind him to take his pills at night?"

"He has his own system for remembering his pills," I tell her, "and I'll call him."

"And so will I," Nic promises. "We'll take care of him."

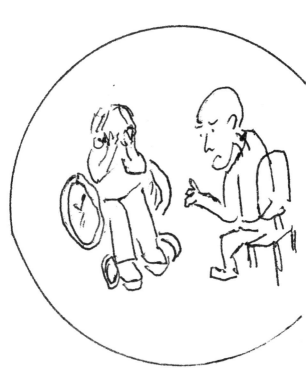

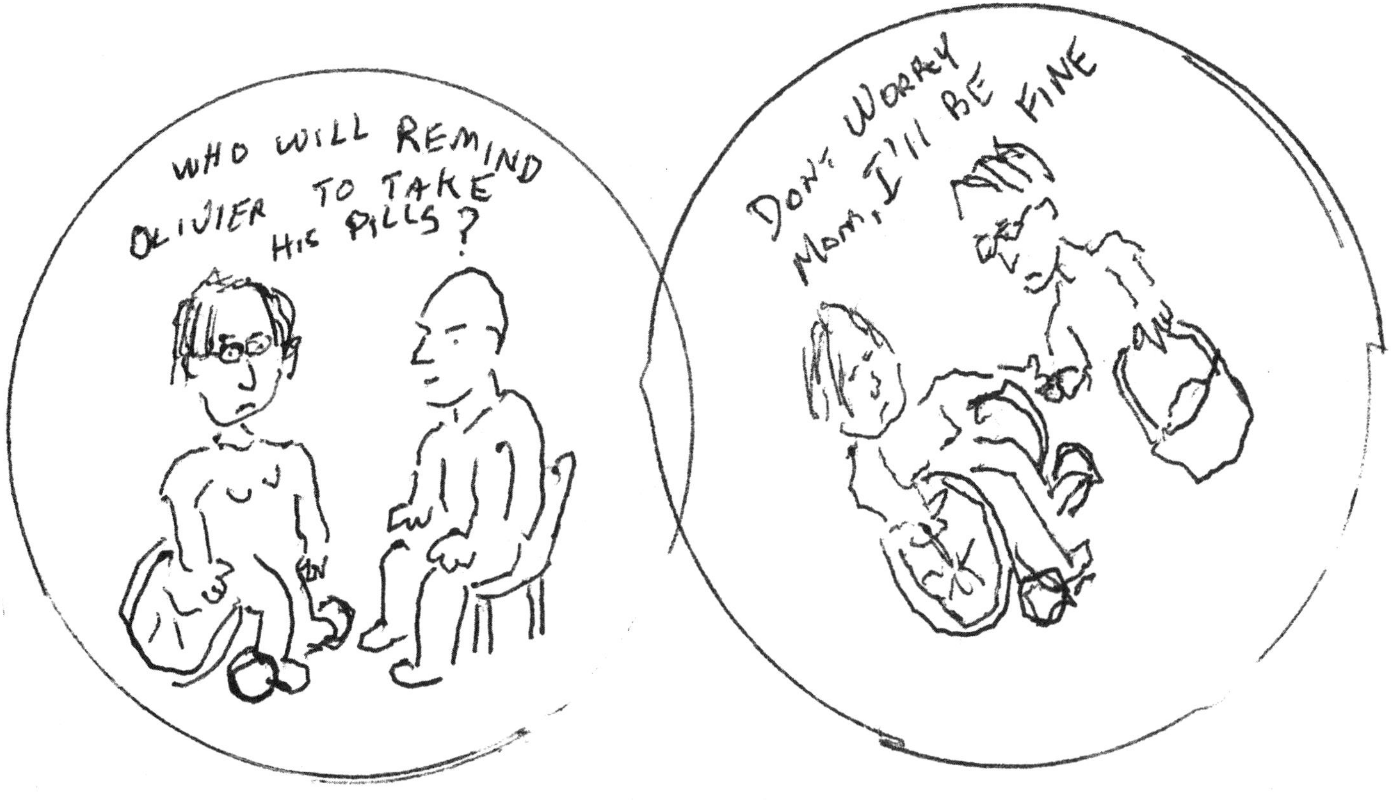
WHO WILL REMIND OLIVIER TO TAKE HIS PILLS?
DON'T WORRY MOM, I'LL BE FINE

Her crying slows. She drops her hands from her face. I pass her a Kleenex. "I've tried to be a good mother," she says as she wipes her nose.

"We know that," I tell her, "we all know that. This isn't about being good or bad, or succeeding or failing. It's about aging and a really unfair disorder."

Our exchange is painful, raw, and frankly without much comfort. But at last we are all able to acknowledge the situation. She nods off, her face finally relaxing and shedding layers of resentment, suspicion, and grief. I pull the sheet up under her chin and watch her as she sleeps, and we camp the night in this last temporary shelter. At 4:00 a.m. we're told that it may be several hours yet until a bed is ready, and I urge Nic to return home and get some rest before he has to be at work. At 6:00 a.m. a bed opens on the seventh floor. An orderly transfers Mom on a rolling metal gurney to a small, shared room in a ward for elderly patients. We slip past her new roommate, who lies stiff as a fallen tree atop her bed, her head craned to one side, her mouth gaping. The room is still except for the rhythmic gasping of her neighbour. My mother sits upright on her bed, her hands folded on her lap, and stares out the west-facing window.

The sun rises after the long night, mountains glinting like teeth in the distance, a jagged line of rusty peaks cloaked in a dark bank of clouds. Wind abruptly gusts, rattling the window with tiny, hard pellets of snow.

"It will be a cold day," she whispers.

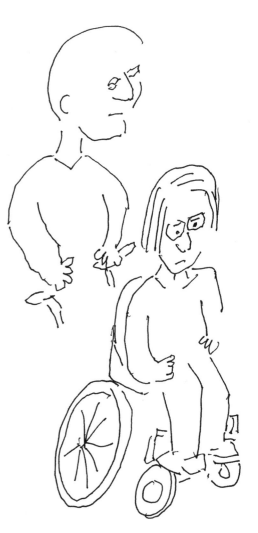

I'm exhausted when I return home, collapse into bed, and sleep for twelve hours, but the following morning Nic and I rise early to hold a cleaning party at Olivier's. We throw open the windows of the apartment and prop the balcony door ajar. Nic fills a rug-cleaning machine with detergent and fires it up. I pitch old materials out, scrub counters and tabletops, mop the kitchen floor, gather garbage bags full of debris, toss dirty clothes in the washer. We drag Mom's mattress from her bed, tip it up, and toss it out.

By the end of our session, the place still needs attention, but the odour is significantly diminished. Liv's bedroom continues to be a huge problem, piled high with discarded clothes, old papers, stale-dated coupons, and general detritus, but it will have to be another day's project.

When I leave Olivier, he has positioned himself on Mom's old chair, looking out the same window at precisely the same landscape as my mother did only days ago.

I LOVE YOU
I LOVE YOU TOO

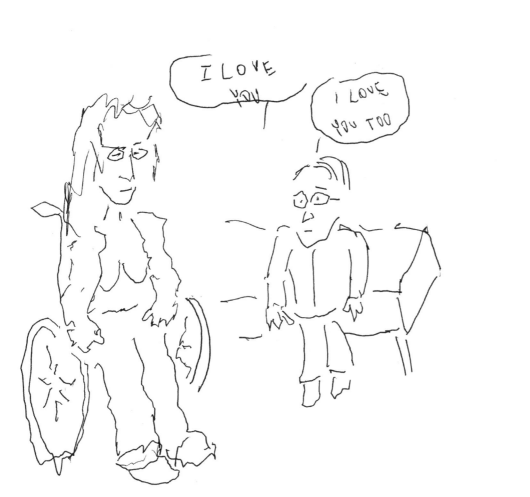

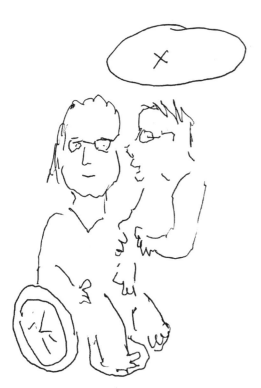

The majority of patients on my mother's floor are scheduled for hip or knee replacements or heart bypass operations. Charts and diagrams of these procedures dot the walls of the corridors — joints separated and labelled, valves being cleansed of constricting plaque. There are a sprinkling of dementia cases on the ward as well; signs warn visitors that the doors at the ends of the hallways are secured to impede wandering patients.

The first few days of hospital life are relatively uneventful. My mother enjoys a better diet than at home. The initial trauma of her intake fades, and is replaced, I think, by a minor sense of calm and relief. Her neighbour doesn't offer companionship, but doesn't trouble her either. Mom passes the time browsing magazines and inaccurately filling out crossword puzzles.

By the third day, though, she's angry, bored, and restless, and doesn't want to stay any longer. My visit coincides with Olivier's, but she initially ignores me, and then turns on me.

"Look at him," she says to Olivier while gesturing at me, "always acting like he's doing something for someone else. He pretends to care, but he only cares for himself."

I'm not sure how I should respond. "That's pretty mean," I tell her.

She shrugs. I guess she intends it to be.

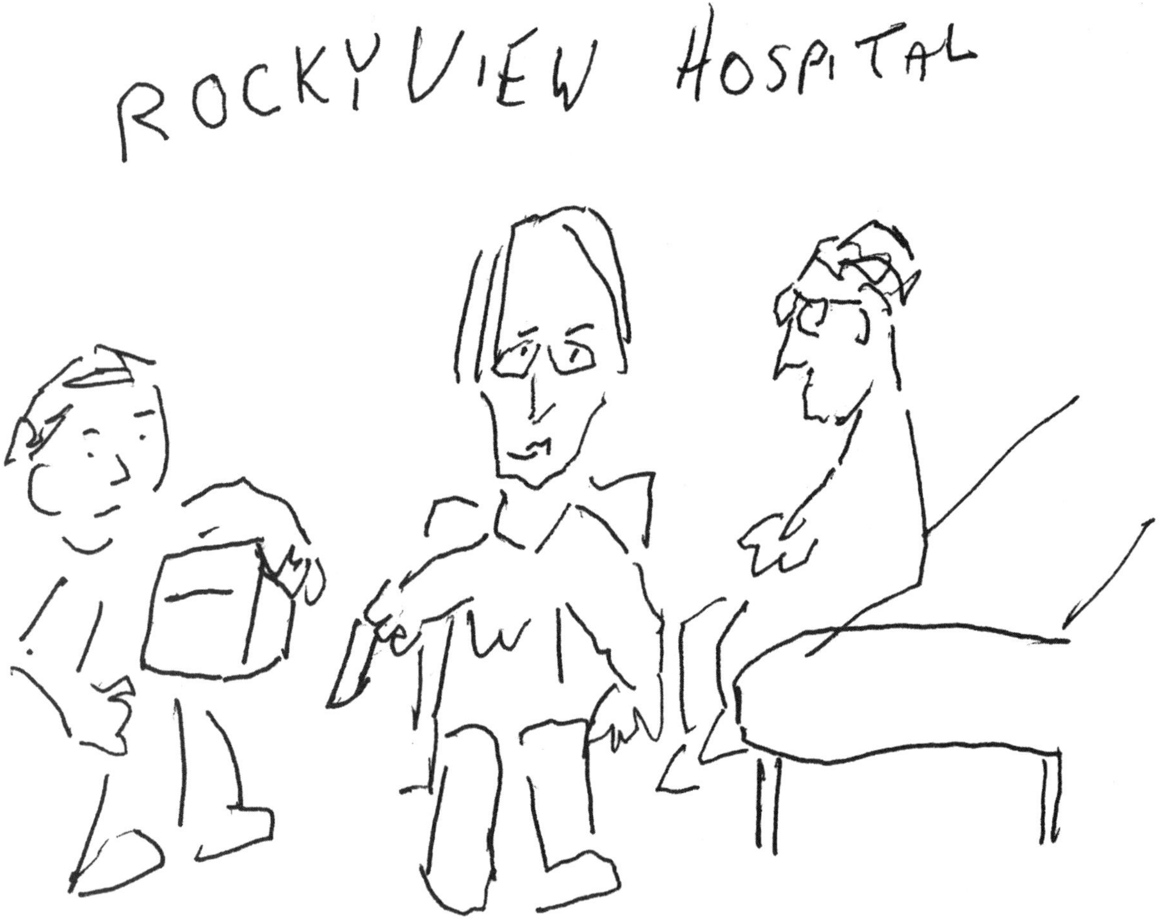
ROCKYVIEW HOSPITAL

Above the cliffs rising along the Glenmore Reservoir, in the south end of the city, sits the Rockyview Hospital. When it was first constructed, the building seemed elegant and new — a castle. Now it operates beyond capacity and odd Lego-like trailers and temporary units have been attached, giving the facility a ramshackle, derelict appearance.

Like all the hospitals in the province, it claims to have a no smoking policy. Large signs posted at each doorway announce that smoking is not permitted on any portion of the hospital property. Immediately opposite the signs, patients — many of them hooked up to IVs — lounge in wheelchairs and defy the ban, smoke coiling above their heads in grey-blue clouds.

The transition unit, where my mother is transferred after six days on the seventh floor, is wedged into a neglected corner of the hospital, accessed by a single, ancient, slow-moving elevator. As soon as the elevator door gapes onto the fourth floor, you are confronted by the unsettling odour of pureed food, stale urine, and bleach.

The aged residents of the unit pass the time seated and still, confined in the chairs of their shared bedrooms or parked in wheelchairs along the narrow hallway.

On Mom's first day we're informed that the transition unit is a hospital service, not a seniors' care facility. Clothes aren't washed and disposable undergarments won't be provided — that will be our responsibility. As Mom spends more time here we also learn that there will be no genuine attempt to forge relationships between staff and patients. Relationships are what occur when people stay in one place, and the guiding principle of this unit is to keep patients moving. A whiteboard tacked up across from the check-in desk details incoming and exiting patients, like the flight chart at airports. A few organized activities are sketched onto the whiteboard — singalongs and wheelchair calisthenics — but patients tend not to participate. Meals are served in a kidney-shaped bend in the hallway where patients are first herded, then seated and penned in by heavy plastic tabletops clamped atop their chairs. There they wait for their meal trays to be distributed from a stainless steel food trolley; once finished eating, they wait again for staff to detach the tabletop. They are then free to straggle back to their rooms to continue what seems to be their only real activity: waiting.

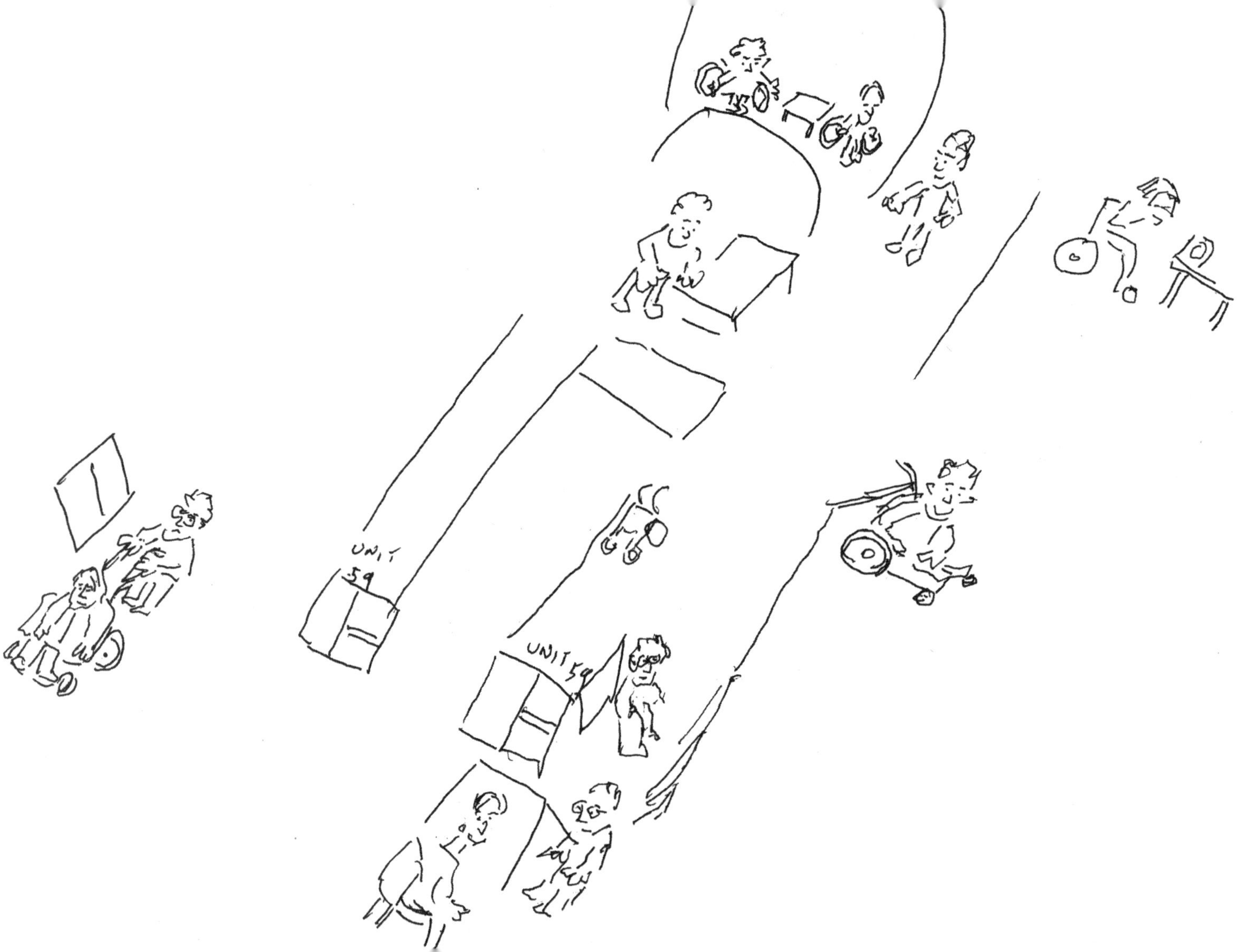
UNIT 59
UNIT 59

As the weeks pass I become increasingly appalled by the level of indifference on the unit — the lack of human contact or supervision, the perfunctory manner in which the elderly patients are cared for.

It's hard not to see this as an extension of how the aged are viewed in our culture. They are shoved to the edges of everything. Newspapers rage that the elderly stay too long in their jobs, clinging to positions that the public feel rightly belong to younger employees, then fume that those who do retire and collect pensions are a drain of the public purse. At the point in their lives when they most need medical assistance, they are viewed as a burden on health care — and a growing one, a threat to the national economy.

It's a tidal wave, we're told, a *tidal wave* that will displace the industrious young and healthy.

The tone of these public discussions is remarkably similar to the tone adopted when discussing the mentally ill, who are frequently viewed as slackers, or worse, parasites. After all, *everyone* feels depressed sometime, everyone gets a little confused — but they don't demand a handout.

Those who are old and mentally ill get the worst of both worlds. Because they are expensive to care for and viewed as incurable, they are placed in large segregated institutions that are essentially holding tanks for those who suffer from Alzheimer's and other neurological disorders. Since they can't be cured, we're told, it's best to put them someplace safe and out

of the way. And perhaps that's true. But one should remember this was precisely the same rationale which precipitated the emergence of the immense, and immensely damaging, psychiatric institutions that thrived right up through the seventies, leaving a horrifying legacy of forced labour, willful neglect, and sexual and physical abuse.

Many things slip my mother's mind, but not her birthday. February 27. As the day approaches, she reminds me repeatedly that "turning ninety isn't something you do every day."

The entire extended family convenes for the event, bearing cake and drinks and presents. The celebration convenes in the small, rather nondescript meeting room that we're permitted to use at the end of the hall. Mom wishes to dress up and arrange her hair for the event. I've brought a brush, hairpins, and several outfits for her to choose from.

As she readies herself, she displays her best and worst behaviours: rejecting every offer of help from the hospital staff and trying their patience, shouting, nearly collapsing several times, losing things and fuming about it; then once she is ready, thrusting her walker through the hallway like it is a carriage conveying royalty. Entering the meeting room, she makes a point of recollecting Cheryl, and Nic's wife, Marg, and all the grandchildren, Ben and Ian, Naomi and Kimi, Chandra and Miranda, and inquiring of them individually. We sing "Happy Birthday" to her. She nearly expels her dentures extinguishing the candles, eats her cake, and is happy. She's made it to ninety.

It's a pretty good show. It's equally, I understand, an act of defiance intended to demonstrate that she doesn't truly need to be in the hospital.

The following morning I pop by Liv's and discover the apartment has taken an unfortunate step backwards. Dirty dishes, opened food containers, and plastic wrappers cover the kitchen counter and liberally dot the living room. Dirty clothes collect in crumpled piles on chairs, the sofa, the floor. The television is busted — it has been malfunctioning for months and has apparently finally given up. Liv sits in front of it, staring absently, with the appearance of being immobile.

I tidy up around him and ask how he's feeling about remaining in the apartment on his own. Eyes still fixed on the darkened television screen, he says he's coping, then confesses that he feels lonely without Mom and that the evenings are hard. I remind him he doesn't have to stay on his own: we can explore a different solution. He says he'd like to try a while longer to see how he manages.

I worry that he's ruminating — returning to a single troubling thought and turning it over obsessively. It's a characteristic of his schizophrenia — and without someone to share the apartment, without even the presence of a television to distract him, he may spiral down. In the past, ruminating has precipitated his breakdowns.

As a stopgap, I urge him to scan the flyers for a new TV. He nods distantly, his thoughts elsewhere. While I secure and place garbage bags by the door, I suggest that it might be worthwhile for the three of us brothers to sit down together the next time he meets with his psychiatrist. Maybe we could talk a few things through. He brightens, says that sounds like a good idea, and tells me he'll bring it up with Dr. Baxter at his next appointment.

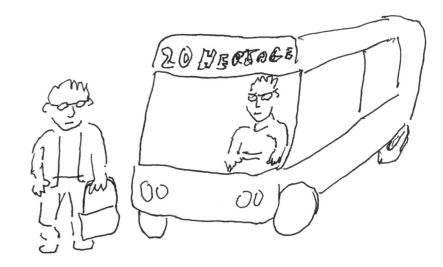

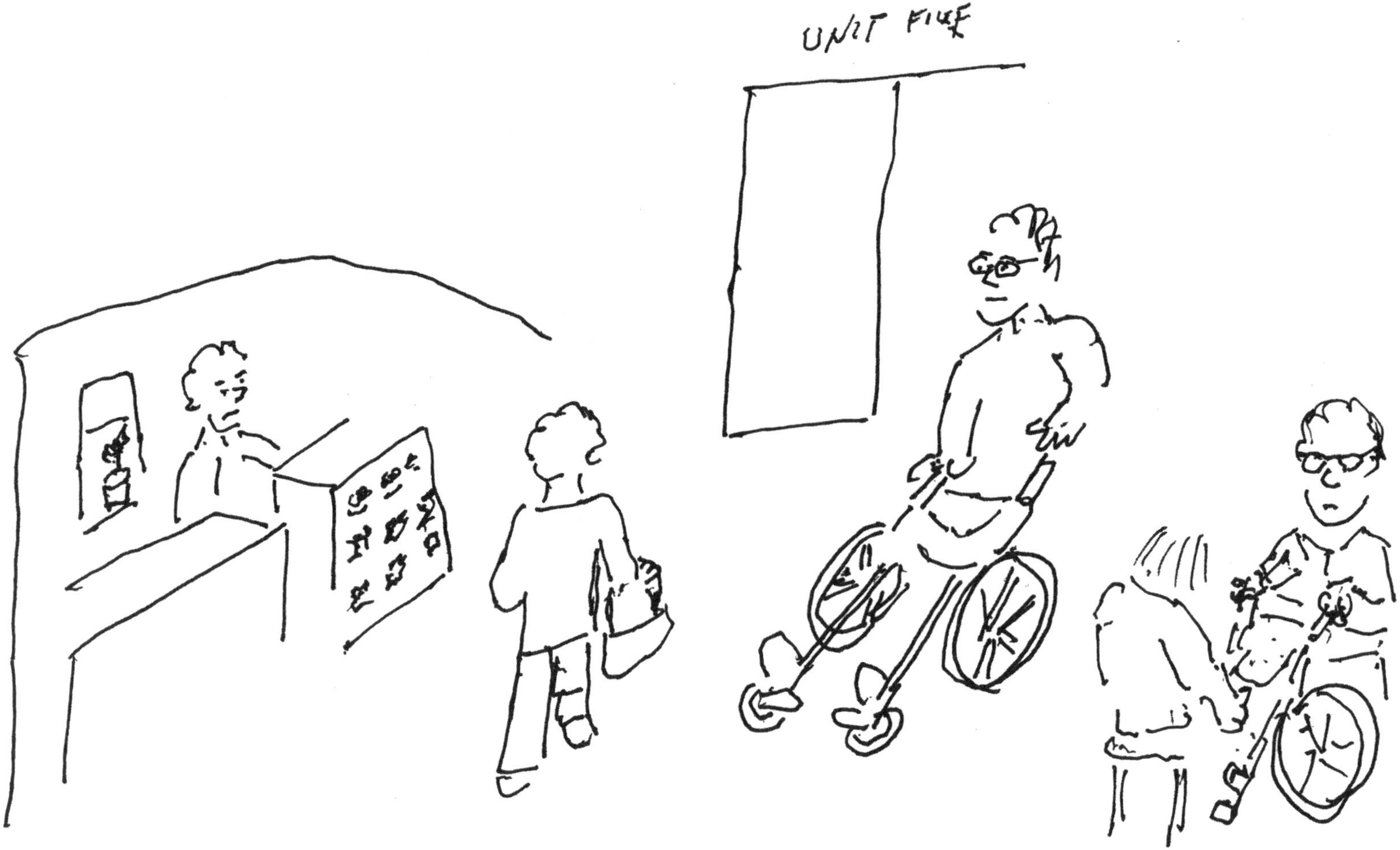
UNIT FIVE

I draw up a chair beside my mother, who's crammed into what has become her new usual space – seated between the bed and the wall, behind the door – filling in crossword puzzles. I've brought chocolate and mandarins to share. As we snap the chocolate into squares and peel the oranges, we chat and I remind her that medical personnel will be applying tests over the next weeks, this time to determine the kind of facility she should attend. She rolls her eyes in response, and mutters, "More tests. Goody."

I place a hand on her shoulder and urge her to be patient, and not shout or argue or get angry. The sooner they complete the assessment, the sooner she can move to a better facility.

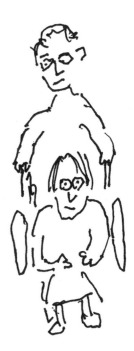

She's piled the cold remains of her dinner to the side of her bedside table, making the confined space of the room feel even more crowded. When I ask why she won't eat in the hallway with the others, she makes a face. She tells me that once there, she must remain seated until a nurse comes to release her. That can be a lengthy operation and she gets cold waiting. The hospital staff have taken to dressing her in hospital garb to facilitate taking her to the washroom. The gowns are flimsy and her legs are bare.

She complains that it's been a long time, and she puts particular emphasis on the word *long*, since she had any visitors. I remind her I stopped in just a day ago, and both Nic and Liv have been by since then. She shoots a skeptical glance at me, but I've come equipped. I pull a notebook out of my backpack and place it on the bedside table. I write her a message and date it, so she'll know when I last visited, and tell her that all her visitors will sign it, so that she will know who has stopped by, and when. She'll be able to write messages as well, or consult the book when her memory fails.

She briefly acknowledges the book, but continues her original thought, maintaining that she's not surprised that she hasn't seen anyone, because hospital staff actively screen her guests. Surprised, I ask what gives her that impression. She says she can hear them outside her door, in the hallway, warning visitors off. She adopts a gruff voice in a supposed imitation of staff: "No, Mrs. Martini can't see you today."

I tell her that's never happened — not to me, and as far as I know not to Nic or Liv — but she insists that it occurs all the time. She confides that she's even caught the nurses in the act.

"How?" I ask.

She says she looks down — and she demonstrates by glancing downward — and can see staff at the front door to the hospital, extending their arms, and barring the way.

I don't bother replying at this point. She's on the fourth floor and would have to possess X-ray vision to do what she's describing, would have to peer through the bricks, girders, plaster, and paint of the entire hospital to the main entrance located on the opposite side of the hospital.

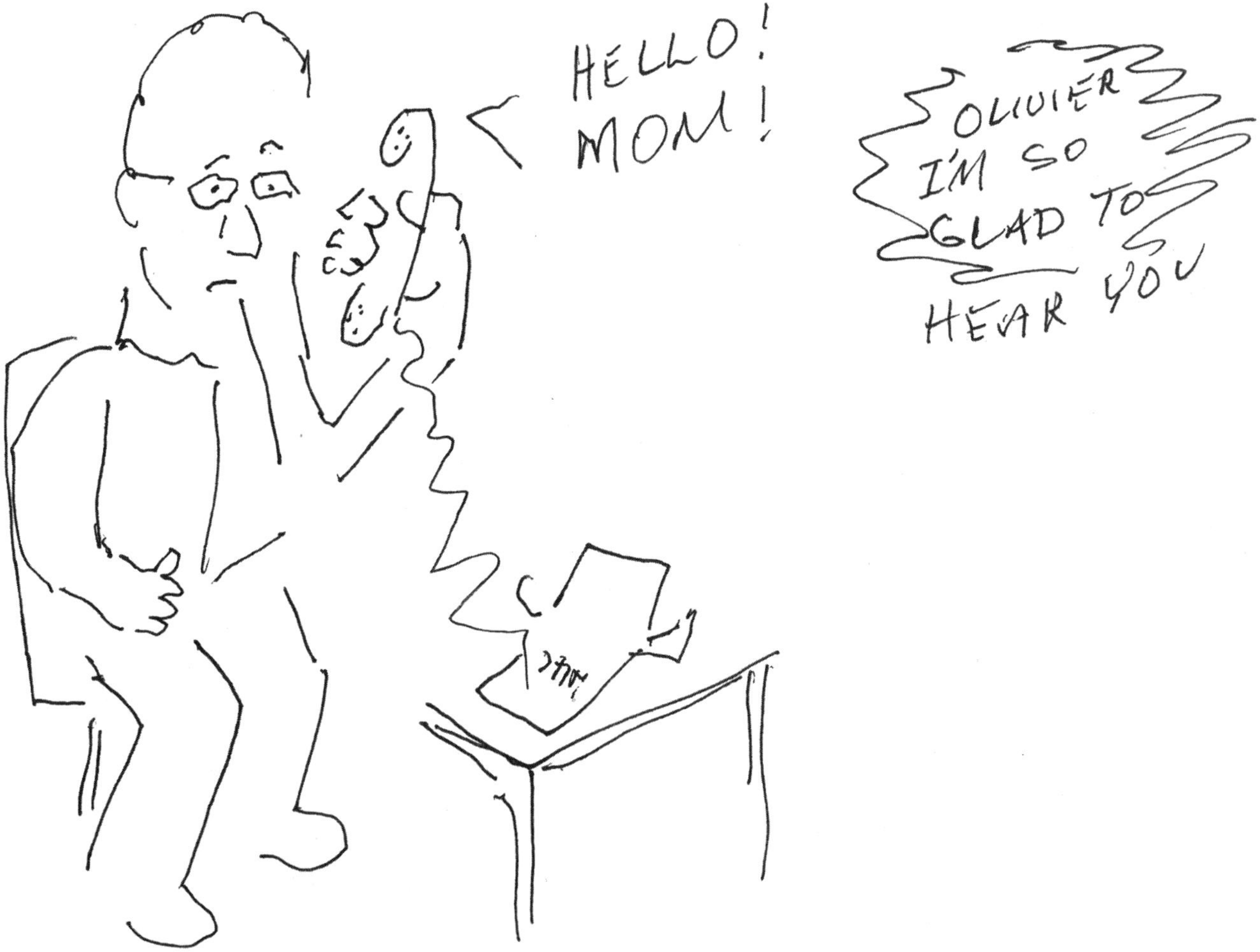
HELLO! MOM!
OLIVIER I'M SO GLAD TO HEAR YOU

In my dream I am lying on my side in a bed. The room is dark and cool — I'm comfortable but I don't recognize this space. It's small and a row of lockers lines the wall. Three men enter without turning on any lights and start unpacking. I think that I must be in a hostel of some kind, that other guests have arrived late. Then one of these men turns on a small flashlight, and I realize they are members of security — or maybe firemen. They are wearing some kind of uniform or overalls.

They turn to me and two of them sit — on benches maybe? — and ask how I am. Only then do I realize that over my blanket there are thick, leather restraining belts. I am fastened in. I tell them I'm fine, but I don't know where I am.

"Do you know why you're here?" one of them asks.

I reply that it must be because of something I did, dangerous or illegal, but I don't recall which. We know, one of them says — he doesn't sound threatening or angry, just matter-of-fact.

"Shall I show him?" he asks.

The others agree, and they turn on a screen, showing video footage that I assume will demonstrate how I have offended. That's when I wake up.

I lie there, in my bed, for some time after, waiting for my crime to be revealed.

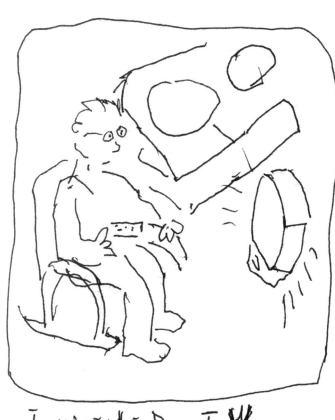

I WATCHED TV

I drive by Olivier's place and pick him up, and together we venture to London Drugs. He's lived without a television for weeks and though I've pointed out that he can probably pick one up relatively inexpensively at a variety of stores, the decision-making process seems to paralyze him.

The electronics section at London Drugs features an entire wall of flickering televisions. Olivier scans the selection and chooses the very cheapest, a black, compact, flat screen RCA, on sale for one hundred dollars. We toss it in the car and bring it back to the apartment. It's a bit of a wrestle hooking it up — there's never anything as simple as plug and play anymore — but twenty minutes or so later it's working. The previous TV was an ancient, hefty vacuum tube model, so this latest purchase features technology new to Liv and represents a bit of a learning curve for both of us. We perform a clinic on how to operate the two remotes required to communicate between the television set and the cable box, then I hand it off to him to try. He turns it on, switches channels, raises and lowers the volume — success! We joke that he is no longer a hermit but is instead magnificently connected to the world once more. *Jeopardy, Wheel of Fortune, The Simpsons, News at Eleven* — nothing is beyond him!

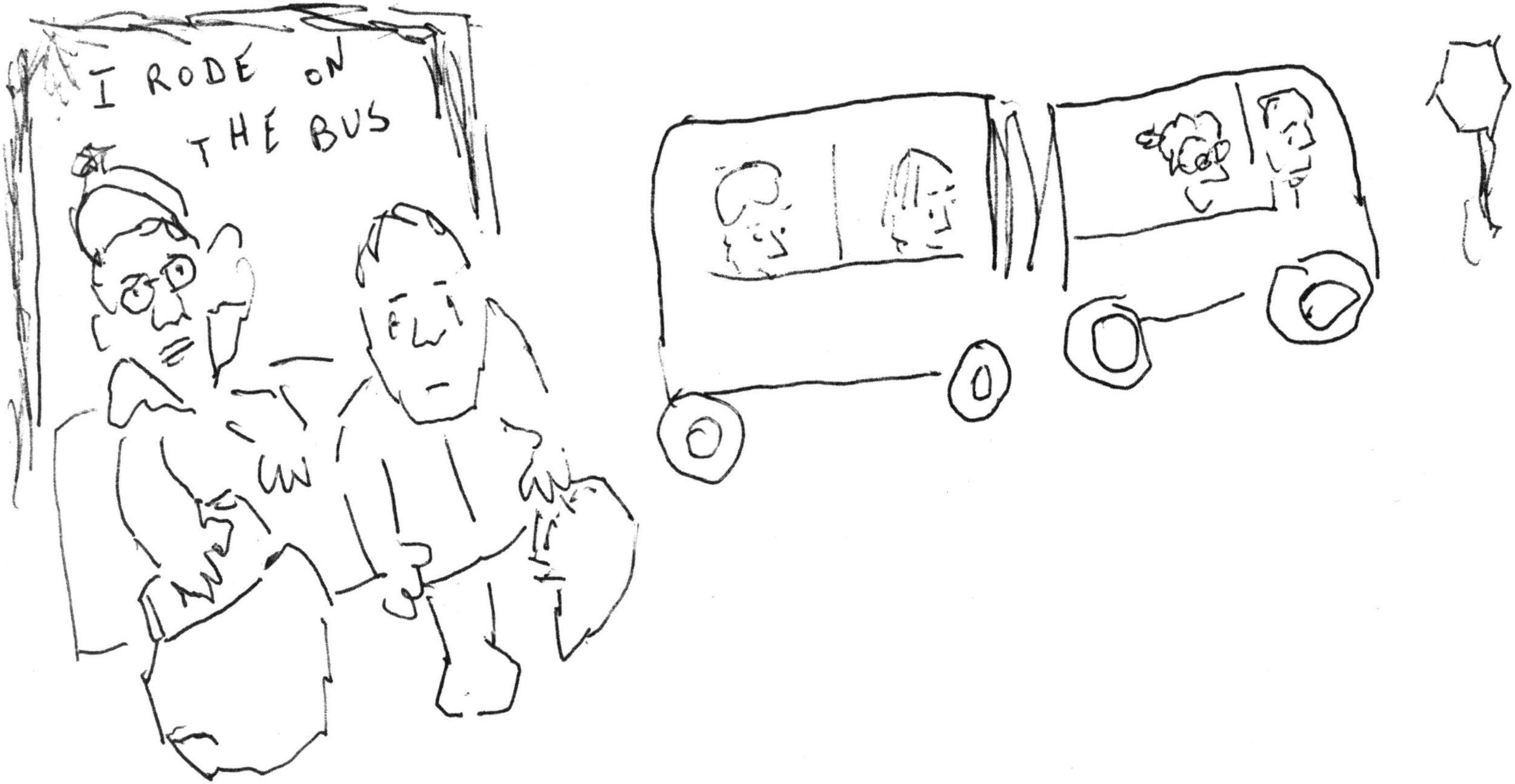
I RODE ON
THE BUS

I call Transition Services, but instead of being put through to the person I've dealt with in the past, am transferred to someone named Trudy. Trudy says that in the future, if I have any questions about Mom's transition, I should speak to her, not Claire. Trudy is handling my mother's file, not Claire, and her tone seems to imply that I've tried to pull a fast one by attempting to get around her. I find the attitude a little unsettling, but apologize and explain that I was just trying to follow up with the person I last talked to.

Trudy says that while it's taken a few weeks longer than planned, our mother's assessment has been completed and her need for Designated Supportive Living (DSL) confirmed. Shortly, we'll be sent a longlist of eligible facilities, and once we have selected our shortlist from that longlist, and delivered our shortlist to the Transition Services offices, my mother's name will be entered into the system. Following that, we can anticipate receiving calls of offer fairly quickly, perhaps within days or weeks. If we haven't heard anything within two weeks, we should contact her.

My mother, Trudy continues, has been ranked SL4, which means she requires assistance with day-to-day decision-making and most/all tasks, and will frequently require unscheduled personal assistance. Trudy reminds me that at government-subsidized SL4 Designated Supportive Living facilities, clients are provided only a shared bedroom and washroom. All furnishings, including a single bed, the accompanying mattress, chair, desk, floor lamp, desk lamp, and anything else my mother might require, must be provided by the client. We should begin assembling these furnishings now in preparation for the move in, because events may advance rapidly.

I'M TIRED

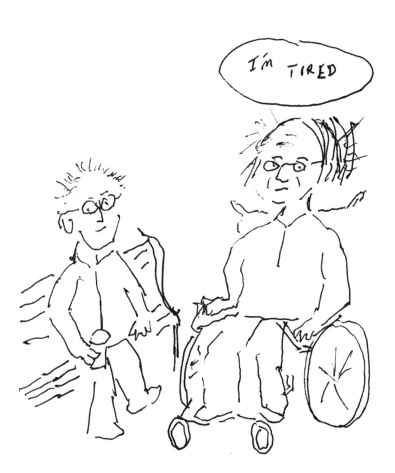

When I return to the Rockyview the next afternoon, I find Mom asleep and seated in a pool of urine. It's seeped through her pad and pants, gathered in her chair, and puddled around her feet on the floor. Her slippers are soaked. I inform the nurse at the desk, who glances up long enough to tell me she'll send someone.

Fifteen minutes later an aide arrives with a mop and bucket to mop up the floor, and a nurse arrives with a clean gown. She draws a curtain, helps my mother change, and scolds her for not letting them know that she needed help. My mother insists she pressed the button.

It's pretty clear to me that no one has been in to check on her for a considerable time, and given that my mother's mental state is as scattered as it is, I suggest to the nurse that someone may want to check in on her more often. The nurse replies shortly that they do check, but there are many patients on the unit.

She reminds me as I'm leaving that we must supply fresh disposable undergarments. I tell her that I'm pretty certain we brought a couple of cartons up earlier this week. After a second look, she finds them.

"Never mind," she says and exits.

The protocols surrounding the selection of a
Designated Supportive Living facility are like
the rules of a complex and not particularly
well-designed board game. First you receive the
longlist of DSL facilities. It's not a full list of the
province's facilities, only partial — selected and
assembled according to some obscure logic.
Why are some facilities included and others not?
Who knows? Why are so many located outside
the city limits, sometimes in distant towns?
A mystery.

From this list, you must choose four institutions, one from your quadrant of the city,
three from outside your quadrant. Once you've
completed this selection and handed it in at the
Transition Services desk, information about the
client is distributed on an electronic list server.

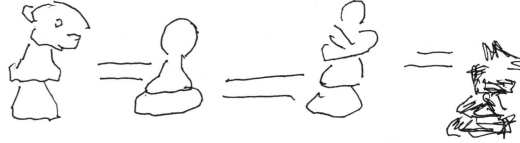

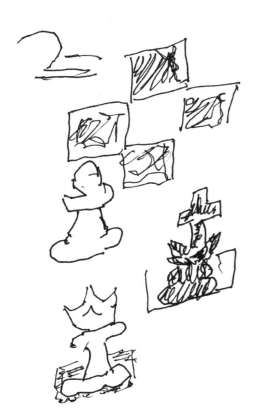

At that point, any facility, on or off the longlist, can make an offer.

If the offering facility isn't on your shortlist, you needn't accept — though you are strongly encouraged to give every offer your most serious consideration. If the offer comes from any of the shortlisted four, you must accept, or get bumped and begin the game again.

Nic and I screen the longlisted facilities, first online, then on foot. Proximity is a critical factor. Driving makes Liv anxious, so mostly he leaves his car parked and relies on public transit. The facility has to be close to a central bus route or CTrain line.

The first facility I check is dreadful in every way imaginable: overcrowded, understaffed, rank-smelling, noisy. The elderly clients cluster in their wheelchairs in the common area, some staring vacantly, some cursing, some weeping or begging for help as I walk by. Some randomly shout. Delusional patients wander the hallways or slip into bedrooms to rifle the belongings of sleeping patients. The few staff present mostly attend to distributing and administering medication. It is an immensely bleak landscape, and I can't help but imagine that if you entered that facility feeling disoriented, frightened, or confused, those feelings would only be magnified.

I leave the facility deeply, deeply discouraged. Obviously, it doesn't make my shortlist, but that it exists at all is depressing.

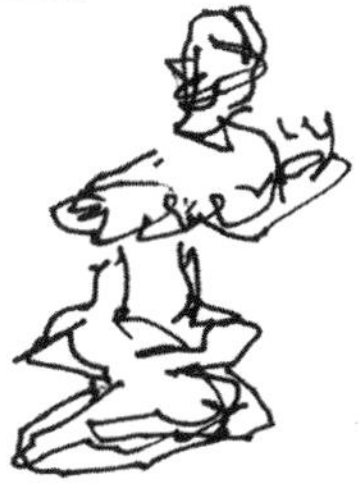

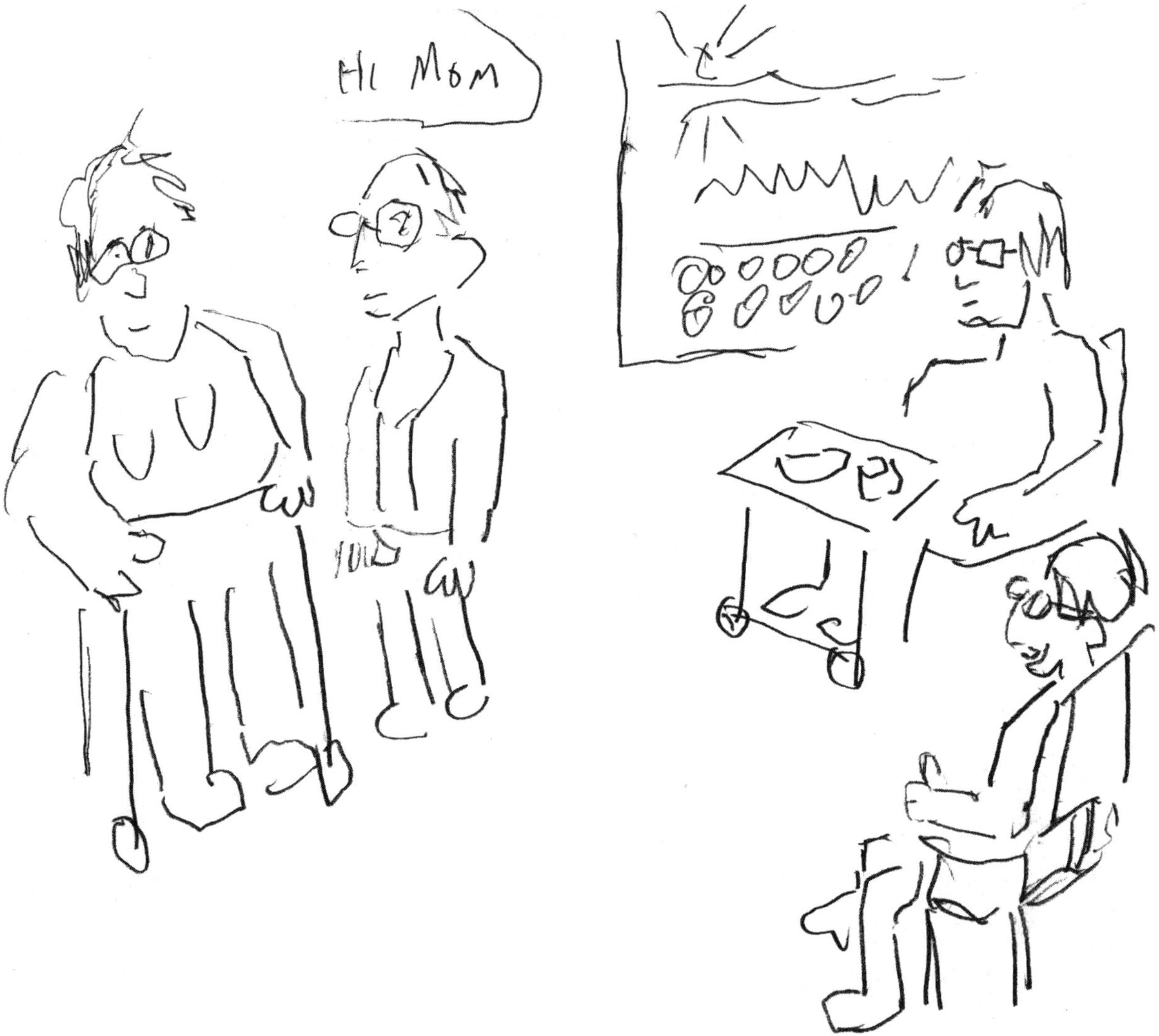
Hi Mom

Three weeks pass without offers. I call Trudy, leave a message. No response. Another week passes.

Every time I visit the unit, and see my mother shoehorned behind the door of her room, see that her dentures have been misplaced and no one has bothered to help her find them, see that a soggy blanket has been folded beneath her chair as a stopgap solution to prevent urine from running onto the floor through her pad, I feel I've betrayed her. Conversations with hospital staff prove fruitless. Nic is stretched thin and spending as much time as he can away from his job and family, as am I. We are doing our best but the fact remains: we convinced our mother to leave her home by telling her that she would be moved to a better place, a safer place, and instead she has been provided three meals a day in a hallway.

I realize that she can't remember the agreement she made, that she was reluctant to make it in the first place, and that if she could recall it now, she would certainly renege. None of that matters. The fact is, we said those words, and she said those words, and together they constitute an agreement, and now I have to find a way to fulfill it. I phone and leave another message with Trudy. Two days later, no reply.

Another week passes and as far as I can tell, transition has ground to a halt.

I send Nic an email, telling him that I'm going to approach some of the supportive living facilities directly. If a space frees up at one institution or another, perhaps a special accommodation can be reached.

There's one, Scenic Woods, that's close to Liv's condo, so it would be easy for him to visit. It offers both private and publicly funded suites. I make an appointment.

A competent, friendly young lady meets me in the lobby, shakes my hand warmly, and leads me on a tour. The facility looks nice — a bit of a cross between a rustic mountain lodge and a spa. An open, airy, wooden-beamed dining area greets you just beyond the lobby.

Further up the hallway a library has been set up with shelves of books and a gas-operated fireplace. Outside, in a flower garden, clients stroll accompanied by staff. The menu for meals changes each day and is posted at the entrance to the dining area. I watch a happy-looking elderly couple drink coffee on the veranda and think what a pleasant change this would be for my mother.

At this point I'm taken to meet with an older individual in the administrative suite who is responsible for client intake. She asks a few questions about my mother, and I, in turn, ask a few questions of my own. How many units are public and how many private? Most are private, she tells me, about eighty percent, but a few units are made available at the lower government-subsidized rate. One of those rooms will be vacated shortly. She takes me to it, and though it's certainly smaller than the private suites, it's comfortable.

I ask how I can get my mother into this room. You can't, she tells me. This room will be allocated "centrally" by provincial authorities and she is unable to tell me who controls allocation, can't predict who will be selected to get that room, and can't offer me any sense of how that selection even occurs. I'm flummoxed. I try to think of another organization with as much mystery attached to its selection process as the province's seniors' care authority, and beyond certain religious cults, can't.

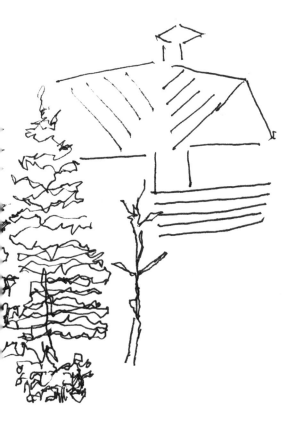

We step out onto the deck overlooking the gardens in the back and I ask if there is anything else available immediately. There is, she tells me — a private room. The private rooms are larger, and cost about two-and-a-half times the government-subsidized rate. Private rooms are assigned directly by the facility and I can have one in an instant. I crunch the numbers. Although the monthly rate wouldn't be financially sustainable in the long run, it could work for the space of a few years. By then, one of the subsidized spaces might become available for my mother through the inscrutable selection process.

I ask to view a private room. It's wonderful: spacious, quiet, with its own washroom and a shared kitchenette. A simple comfortable chair rests in the corner. There's nothing institutional about it — it looks like a small, homey apartment. I'm told that if I wish, my mother could move in next week.

My host conducts me back to her office and explains the terms of the agreement, and I accept them. She smiles and hands me a package of forms. The next step, she says, will be to bring my mother in for an assessment. I'm surprised. Can't they apply the assessment that's already been completed in the hospital? No, she answers, it's necessary that they employ their own in-house procedures. I'm not sure what they will be looking for that has not already been "assessed," but I agree.

"Do you mind," she asks, "if we call the hospital to collect information?"

"No," I answer, "why would I mind?"

I HAVE ANOTHER MEETING SOON
ANOTHER DAY
I'M TIRED

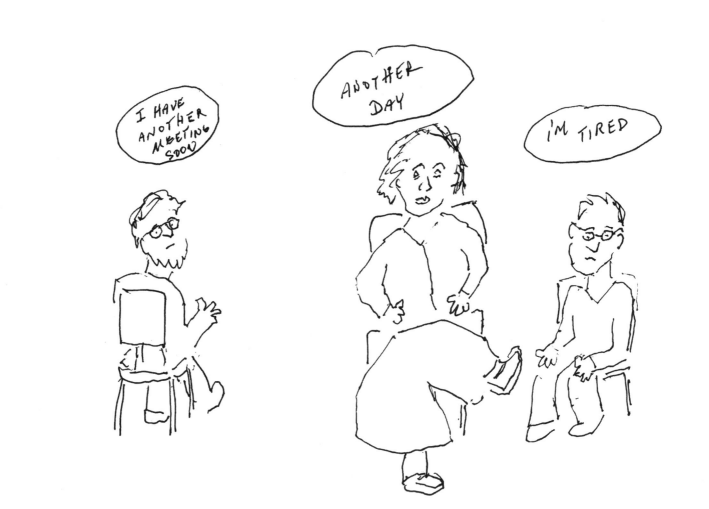

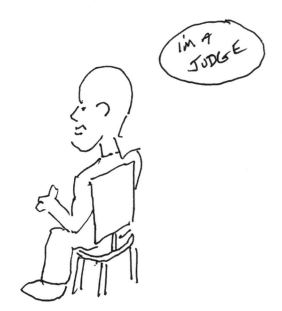

As Nic and I open the door, a quiet electronic chirp announces our entry into the suite of offices that Dr. Baxter shares with two other psychiatrists. We're early for the appointment Liv scheduled, so we sit on the couches provided and wait. Olivier hurries in moments later, carrying a portfolio in preparation for meeting with a member of the Schizophrenia Society who has made an offer to buy one of his paintings. He leans the portfolio against the wall.

Dr. Baxter, an imperturbable woman in her mid-fifties, emerges from a hallway, offers us tea or coffee, then conducts us into a spacious, uncluttered office where four chairs have been arranged in a circle. We sit and she welcomes us, tells us that Olivier expressed an interest in bringing us together to chat about how things are going now that he's living on his own. She turns her attention to Liv.

I've never attended a session with Dr. Baxter and I'm interested to see how she and Liv connect. He's told me in the past how much he admires her, and it's clear from how relaxed he is around her that they have a relationship based in trust.

How does he think things are going, she asks? Fine, he says. Is he eating properly? He assures her that he is. What does he mean, she probes, when he says that he's fine? He tells her he sees friends and attends art classes, has sold a few paintings, recently enrolled in a couple of new social groups, and is participating in a volunteer training group. He exercises regularly at the Y and visits Mom daily.

And what about his evenings, Dr. Baxter asks. Liv shifts in his seat, then admits that he feels at a loss many nights. And his sleep? Mostly okay, though sometimes he finds himself awake late. She returns to his diet. Does he think that he's buying the groceries he needs? He says he thinks so.

She folds her hands on her lap. "What was your dinner yesterday evening?" she asks.

He hesitates. "A couple of bananas."

Raising an eyebrow, she suggests that this isn't sufficient. Because he's diabetic, and because his antipsychotic medication requires that food be eaten along with it, it's critical that he maintain a proper, balanced diet.

Turning her attention to Nic and me, she invites us to share our feelings. We tell her we're just trying to figure out how best to support Liv. Nic points out that Olivier is living on his own for the first time in nearly forty years. Mom prepared the meals at the apartment. She's no longer there. Before dementia struck, Mom used to keep the apartment in order. Again, she's not there. I talk a little about my anxiety that if Liv experiences a relapse, there won't be anyone around to help. I check in with him regularly, but I may not be able to catch it in time if things go bad. He's attempted suicide in the past. Liv holds his cards pretty close to his chest — he never wants to worry anyone. He says he's okay now, but he always says he's okay, even when he's not. I worry that my mother's absence may trigger a breakdown, the same way that my dad's death triggered a breakdown in 1988. I worry that the stress of taking care of the place on his own may in itself be a trigger, just as the stress of his previous job as a shipper/receiver precipitated a breakdown and landed him in the hospital. If problems arise from his medication — and that's happened several times over the years — how will we catch it?

Dr. Baxter returns to Olivier. What does he think — is living on his own likely to be too demanding?

Again he shifts in his seat and says he doesn't know for sure. Sometimes he feels overwhelmed by the challenges, he admits. He feels guilty about Mom. Again, Nic and I assure him that we don't feel he was responsible in any way. Then he says he's worried that eventually

Nic and I will put him in a facility, like Mom. That takes us by surprise, and kind of crushes me. That he believes that Nic and I are planning to pack him off shows how traumatic the recent struggles and upsets have been for him.

That hasn't even crossed our minds, we assure him. His situation is completely different from Mom's. She was getting sicker and sicker, wouldn't accept help, and it was only a matter of time before something tragic happened. If Liv wants to try independent living, we just need to make sure he can cope. As we wind up the meeting, Dr. Baxter asks what we want to take away from this session.

Liv guesses he should set some goals, and try to meet them. Keeping the condominium in order would be one goal.

"Any others?" Dr. Baxter prompts.

He thinks a moment. "Maintaining an exercise routine," he says, "seeing Mom regularly, and establishing a healthy diet."

I say that I still have to know how we can monitor his mental health. It was Mom who called me this last time about his problems with his medication. And Liv wasn't in any shape to use the phone during that previous episode.

I add that I am uncomfortable going over to his apartment and telling him to clean the place up. I want to be his brother, not his boss. I'm concerned that if I start supervising his apartment he'll come to resent me and it will create a barrier between us. If that happens, how will I be able to help?

Dr. Baxter says she'll assign an Independent Living Skills worker to consult with Olivier, and see if that makes a difference. She urges Olivier to be as open with Nic and me as he can be about how he feels, and suggests that we schedule another meeting in six months, this time at Liv's apartment, so that she can measure whether his goals are being met. We could have tea together, she suggests, and smiles at him. I can tell that Liv is nervous about the idea of hosting a tea party at his place, but also a little excited.

I think it's a great idea. More than that, it's one of the few instances in nearly forty years where I've felt included in a conversation about my brother's mental health, and acknowledged for the role our family plays. I leave the meeting feeling curiously buoyant.

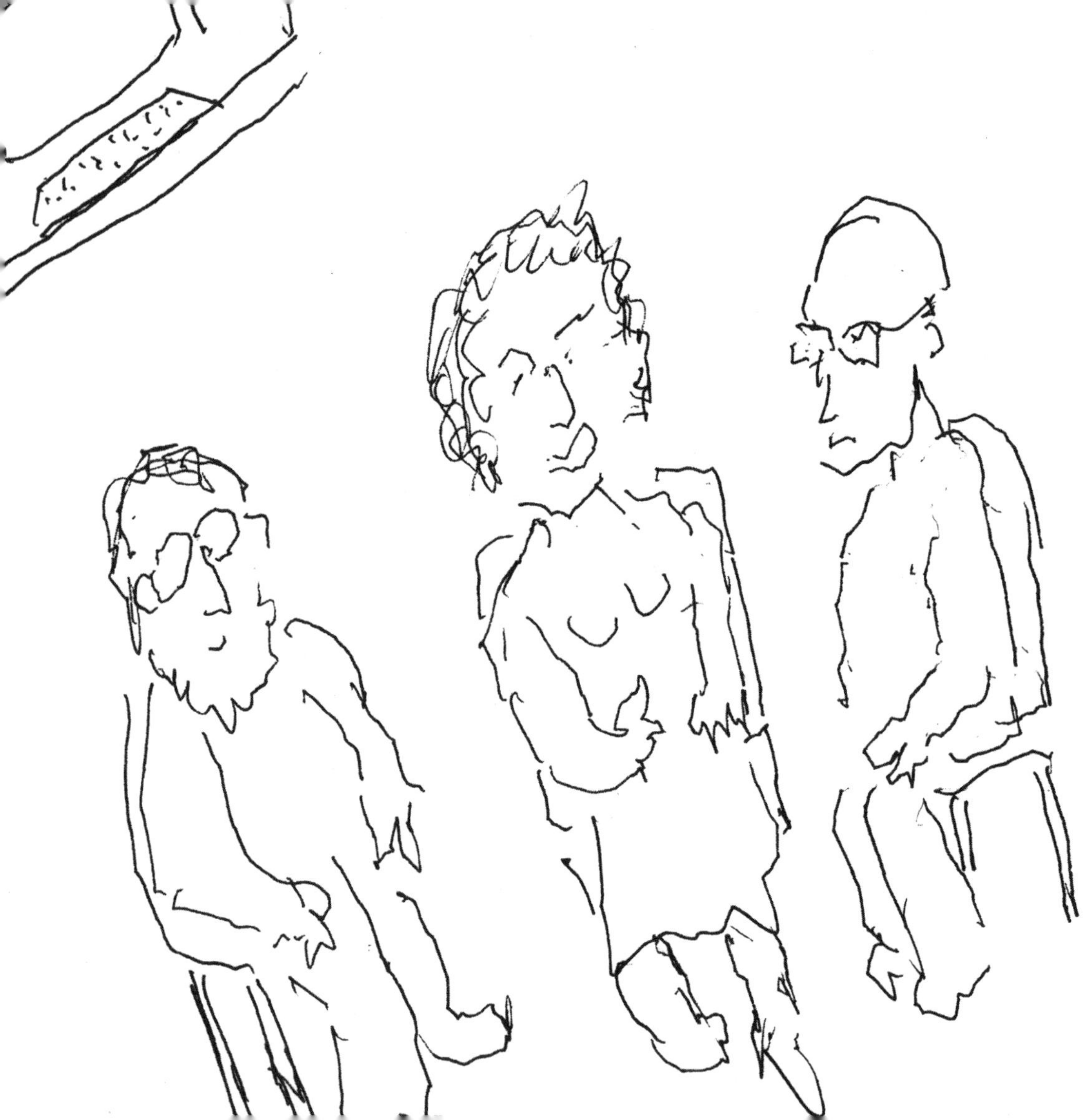

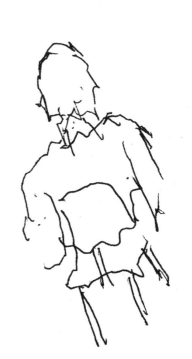

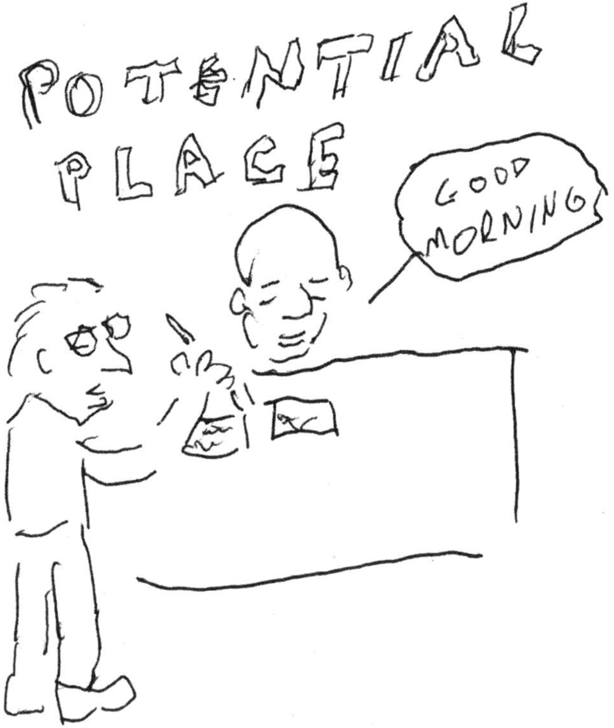
POTENTIAL
PLACE
GOOD MORNING

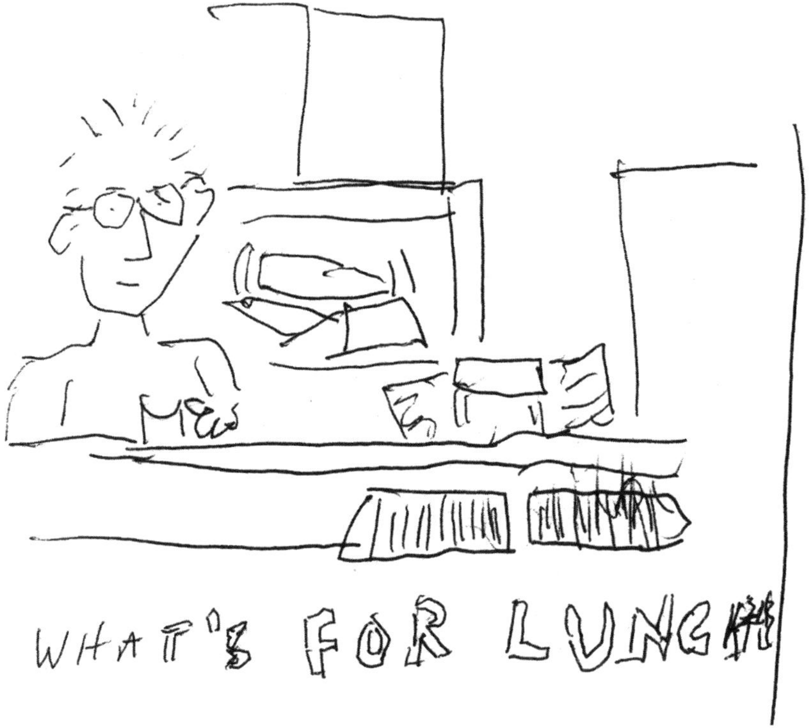
WHAT'S FOR LUNCH

The afternoon before it will take place, I begin preparing Mom for the visit to the supportive living facility. I tell her what will happen, write down in her notebook our departure time. On the day, I sign her out, get her dressed, wheel her down to the car, help her in, and drive her to Scenic Woods.

The moment we get there, I know something is wrong. The treatment by the nurse assigned to assess my mother, while cordial, is completely different to what I received the time before. My mother remains on her best behaviour. The three of us tour rooms and the dining centre, but I can't shake the feeling that we are just going through the motions.

Finally, Mom and I are guided into a meeting room for her assessment. The nurse asks a few generic questions regarding memory, and presents a quick series of pictures that she asks Mom to recall in sequence. My mother, having seen how favourably this facility compares to the transition unit, and desperate to pass the test, becomes anxious that she's being tricked and will fail. "What are you trying to do?" she keeps asking.

The whole procedure takes no more than five minutes, and then, just as it's ending and the nurse is closing her notebook, she asks me, almost as an afterthought, if my mother has bowel incontinence. Surprised at the abrupt change of direction, I answer yes. The nurse makes another quick note, then requests that my mother stand, although surely she must already know that my mother has trouble walking and standing since she arrived in a wheelchair. Mom rises slowly with the usual show of exertion. The nurse says she will take her information to her team to review — but there may be concerns about Mom falling, and adds that the facility isn't really set up to handle bowel incontinence. None of the information she's gathered today is new. She must have been informed at least two days earlier when she contacted the transition unit.

I run my mother back to the hospital and then return home. I've no sooner stepped into the house than I receive a phone call from Scenic Woods informing me that Mom did not pass "screening." I ask what the screening involves, so that I'll know for future reference. She's hesitant to answer at first, but when pressed says that each facility has its own criteria and essentially it boiled down to the issue of incontinence.

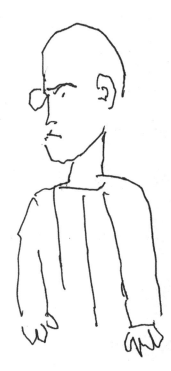

I hang up angry. Why would they put my mother through a strenuous interview, the car ride to the facility, standing up and sitting down, trying to remember their bogus lists and pictures, when from the outset they knew she was incontinent and had already made up their minds? They might have spared us both the trouble and false hope.

But the broader, more frightening implication is that a number of the blended private/public facilities in this province may advertise as being equipped for SL4 Assisted Living (one of the four institutional streams of Designated Supportive Living) but in reality will accept only higher functioning clients. Though they receive government subsidies to build and operate their facilities, and are mandated to serve the public, they keep their costs considerably lower and profits higher by cherry-picking clients who require considerably less care.

When I check the websites of the other private/public facilities on our longlist I discover they all seem to be similarly designed. I suspect we won't be getting any offers there.

When I tell Nic about Mom's interview and her failure to pass inspection, he makes a few quick phone calls to the facilities we've shortlisted and my hunch is confirmed. He is quietly advised that, no, these private/public facilities consider themselves to be operating SL4 "lite" operations and aren't really set up to handle someone with bowel incontinence, so there's no point meeting with them.

I realize that we have to have a frank conversation with the social worker to determine which facilities actually will accept Mom, and then construct a new shortlist based upon this more genuine information. Still more time wasted.

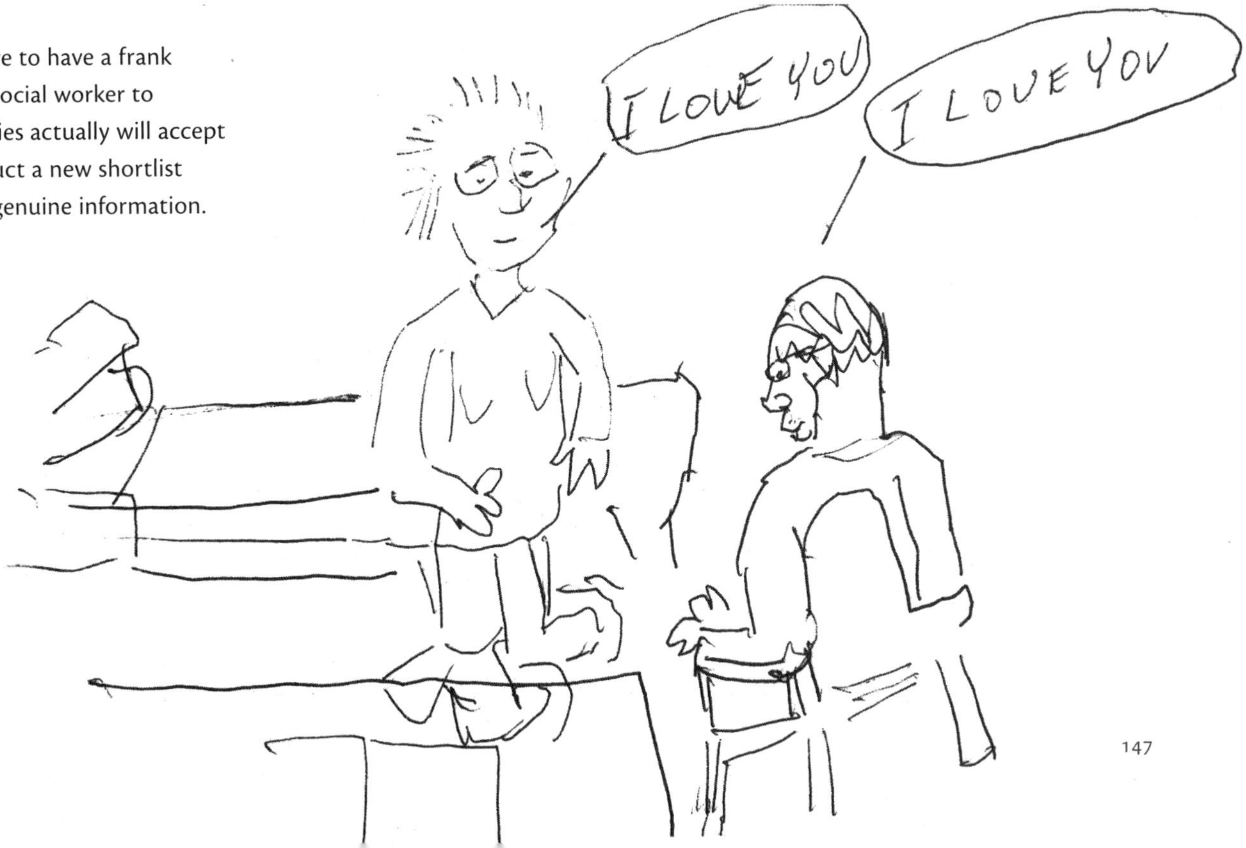
I LOVE YOU
I LOVE YOU

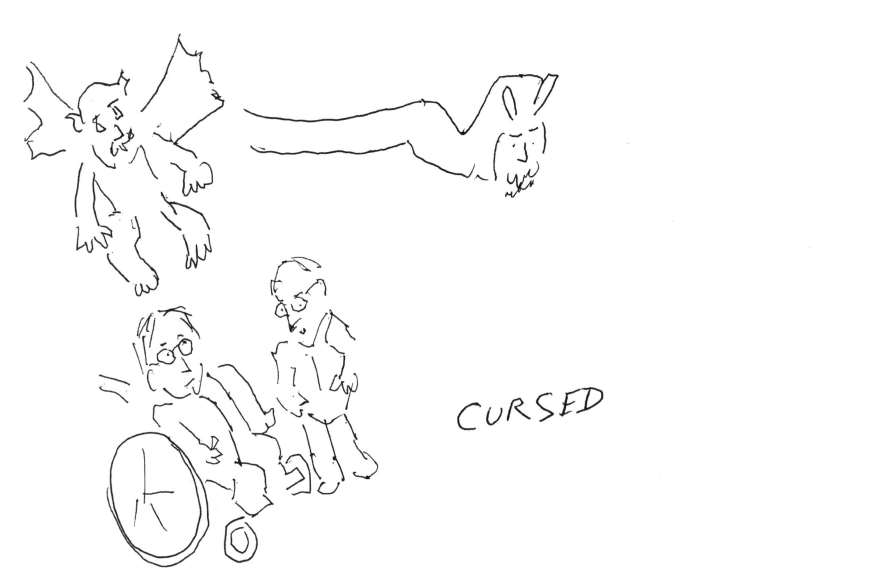

CURSED

At my next meeting with Trudy, her tone alternates between that of a parent addressing a child and an oracle explaining arcane truths to an acolyte. She instantly brushes aside my suspicions about cherry-picking, patiently explaining that every SL4-designated facility — blended private/public or solely public — must accept clients with bowel incontinence.

I tell her I wasn't arguing with her about what was *supposed* to happen, just telling her what was in fact happening. I ask which facilities actually do take clients like my mother. She says they are all supposed to, and offers to send me the list of available facilities. I tell her I already have that list, that my brother and I completed our selection based upon it eight weeks ago — it was delivered to *her* office — but that it is not useful to me anymore if the facilities we shortlisted won't accept my mother.

"What makes you think they won't accept her?" she asks.

"Because," I reply, taking a quick breath and then exhaling to maintain my composure, "they told us they won't, because of her bowel incontinence."

She stops me with a quick admonishing shake of her head. "Every facility with the SL4 designation is supposed to be able to handle incontinence."

"That may be, but they have said they won't. They have told me they won't. And," I add quickly before she can interrupt me once more, "not one has phoned with an offer in months. So can you advise me which facilities *will* take her?"

"I cannot advise you because they are all supposed to take people with incontinence."

"But they don't."

"But they are supposed to."

We stare at each other. "But," I repeat, "they don't." She continues frowning at me, and I'm not sure whether she is considering a further response, or if I have been dismissed.

"What are we supposed to do?" I ask, finally breaking the silence.

"I can refer you to my supervisor if you prefer," she replies.

Inasmuch as her offer to speak with her supervisor sounds more like a threat to be sent to the principal's office than an invitation to get additional assistance, I don't bother taking her up on it.

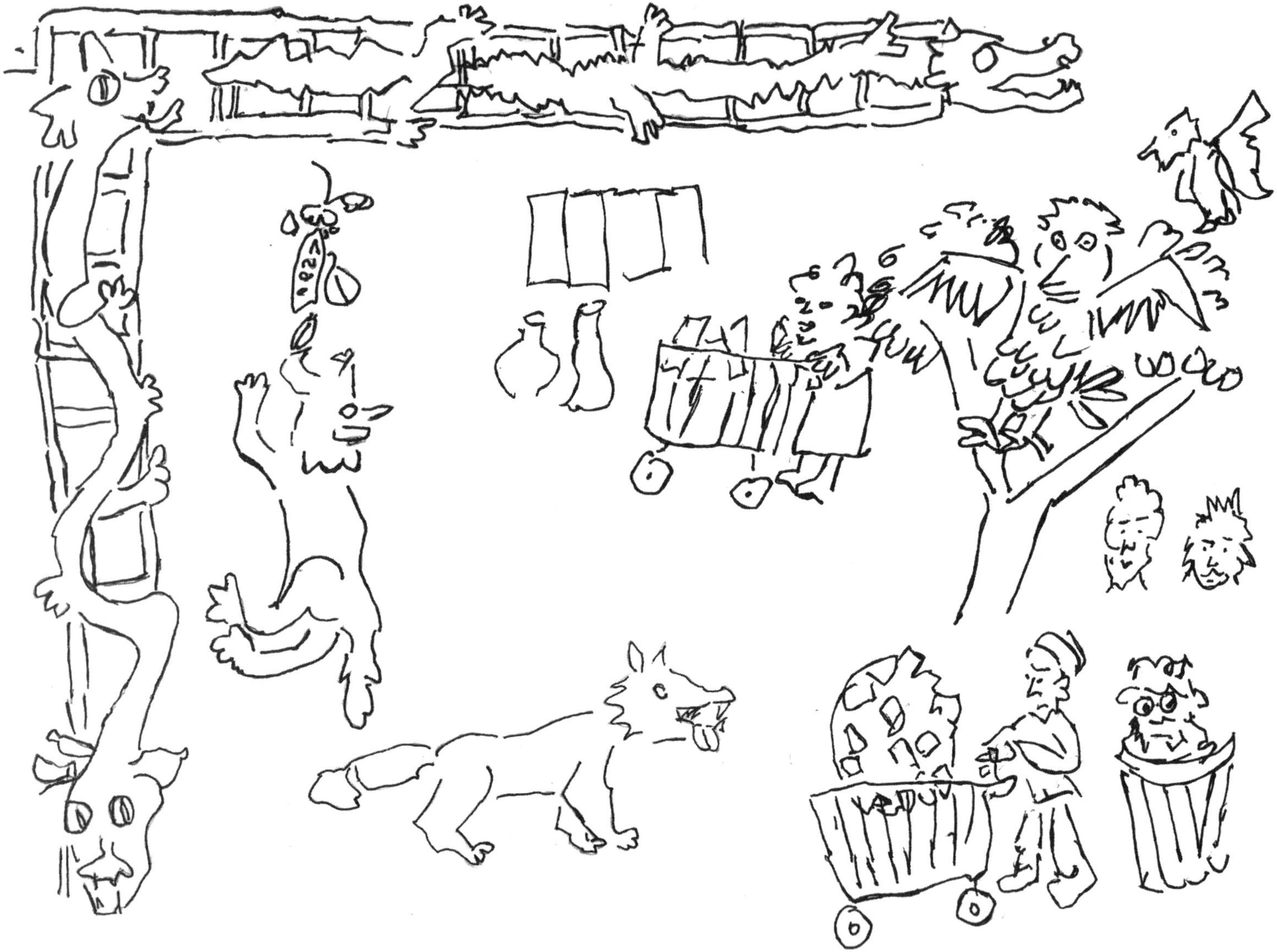

A few days later a phone message informs me that my mother is being reassessed as potentially requiring long-term care. When I visit Transition Services to learn more, I'm told Trudy is out at a meeting and I should leave a message on her cell phone. As I exit the office, I run into one of the two resident doctors who signed my mother's admission to the transition unit. She has stopped in on Mom once or twice to see how she is doing, and I have always found her pleasant.

I ask why Mom is being reassessed. She says she doesn't know, and when I ask what criteria are applied for the assessments in the first place, she says that sort of question is better directed to Transition Services.

I try to frame a question that might help me achieve some clarity, but I honestly don't know where to begin. I tell her I find the structure of Transition Service a bit of a maze.

She nods slowly and says that's a little true for her as well.

So. She smiles sympathetically and, perhaps wishing to end our conversation on a positive note, informs me that if Mom does get assessed as needing long-term care, the upside will be that she should be processed more swiftly. Offering another slight smile of encouragement, she slips away down a corridor.

When I enter Mom's room I find her half dressed in her hospital gown, and looking disoriented. Her glasses have disappeared, and she squints at the menu for tomorrow's meal, which she clutches upside down. I don't think she is aware that she has lost her glasses. I take the menu, turn it right side up, and go through it with her. Together, we mark in her meal selections.

Does she know where her glasses might be, I ask. At this point she actually twigs to the fact that she isn't wearing any. Perhaps on the bed, she suggests. We turn and glance at the bed. Not there. I search the room, eventually finding the glasses under a stack of paper towels in the washroom.

I lean in to slide the glasses back onto her face, then stand and survey the sterile, cramped quarters, and the flickering fluorescent lighting. Her new neighbour, a sad, lonely, withdrawn lady of about the same age as my mother, cries softly behind her drawn curtain. My mother confides with a slight note of irritation that her neighbour spends most of the day doing that. I glance outside, see trees bending in the wind, and reflect that spring has nearly passed.

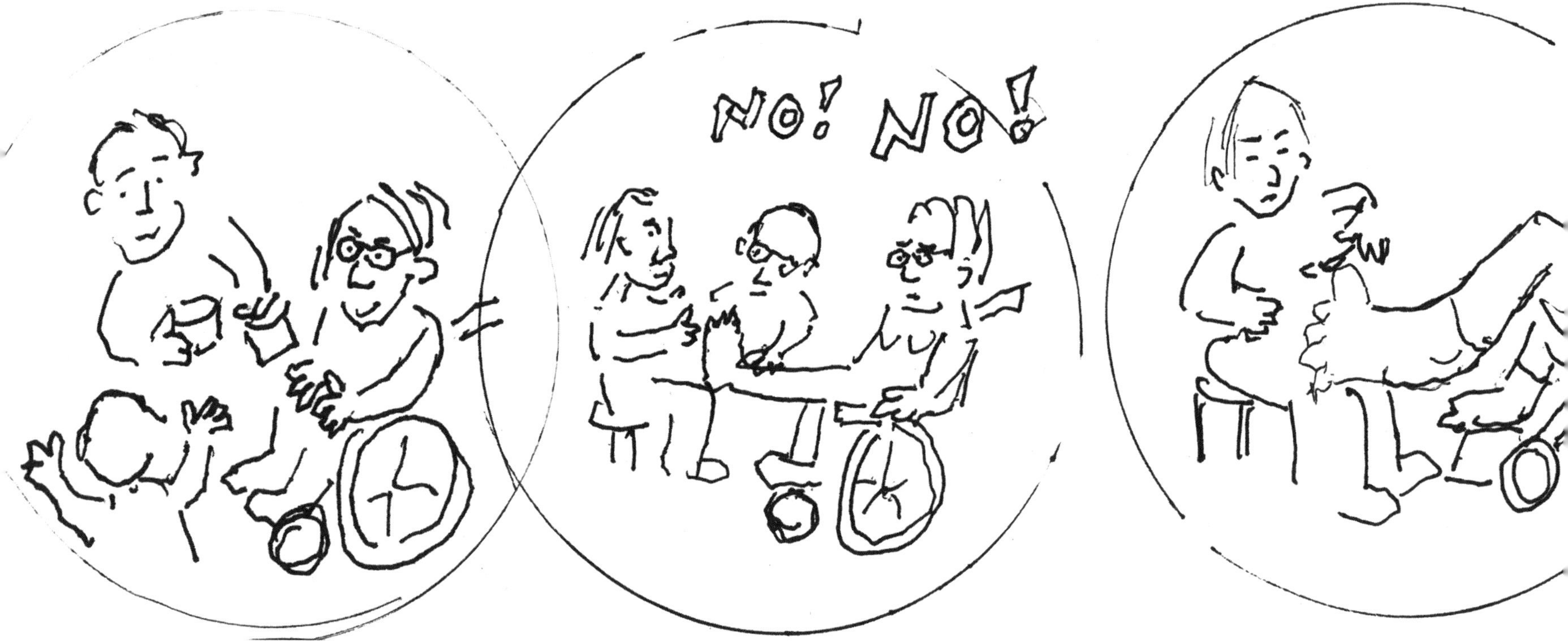
NO! NO!

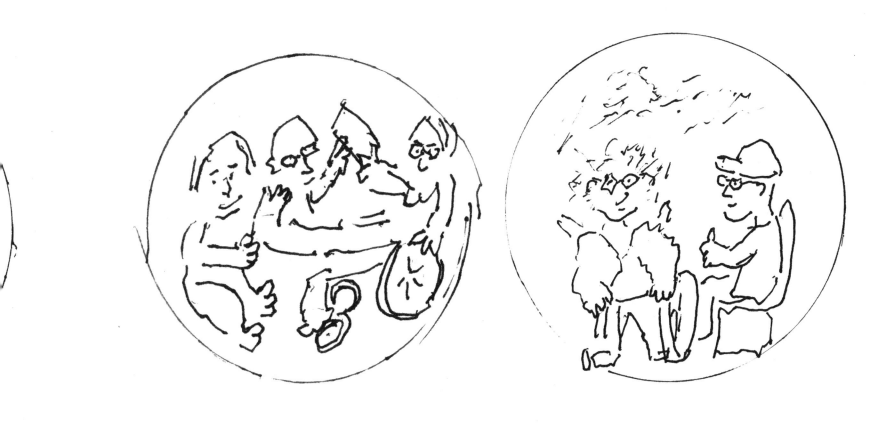

Of course, there's no room for anger or even its weaker cousin, resentment, in any exchange with health authorities, because it's never you that runs the risk of facing consequences. It is always the individual in care who may suffer, and you can never be certain how that will play out. Will my mother be ignored? Will assistance be offered grudgingly? These kinds of things are almost impossible to measure.

And of course, everything is relative. However many elements you may feel are amiss, you will be told you are lucky. Has your mother waited months for a placement – lucky you! There are others who have waited longer. Is your mother in a tiny, dimly lit shared room – how fortunate for you! Others are crammed into rooms with two or three clients and no windows at all. Is the care unfriendly and unresponsive? Lucky, lucky you! At least they're doing something. There are facilities so overburdened that patients are left entirely to their own devices for hours on end, facilities where the staff are so overworked that patients must rely on family to do everything outside the most pressing matters.

Nevertheless, knowing that anger and bitterness are a pointless waste of energy, here are a couple of entries on my growing Go Screw Yourself list.

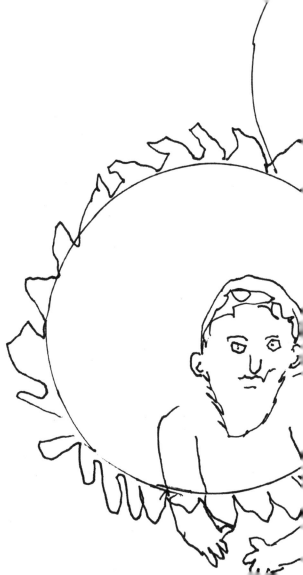

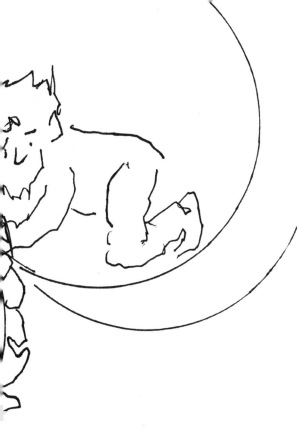

First: the coordinators of a care system for the elderly that is intentionally cryptic, a system that, as it exists now, is no better than a Ouija board that you may consult to little or no effect. How long will it take for decisions to be made? Nobody can say. Who is in charge? Impossible to tell. Who is accountable? A cipher, a will-o'-the-wisp, a phantom. How are decisions arrived at? What criteria and what protocols are used? Nobody in the system, not even the people nominally coordinating the process, can say with any certainty. Well, the engineers of this system — whoever they may be — first and foremost can certainly and most definitely go screw themselves.

Second: the designers of a system of care for the aged that is so obviously skewed on the basis of income can also take their much-deserved place on the list. The most modern facilities are those that, while accepting every available public subsidy, are run for private profit, and the way to make a profit is to turn away the difficult cases. This leaves the solely government-funded care centres to deal with the most challenging clients, often in the oldest, most outdated, most crowded facilities. Those responsible for a system that so blatantly privileges higher-income residents, and punishes lower-income seniors, can most energetically and enthusiastically go screw themselves.

HEY

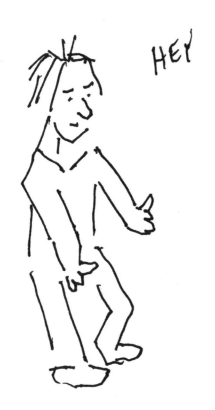

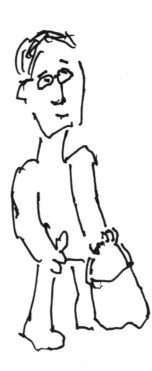

Today, on the phone, Liv asks me out the blue, "Do you think they really hate me?"

"Who?"

"Everyone," he says. "The world."

"No," I answer, puzzled. "I'm pretty sure the world doesn't hate you. Almost everyone I know likes you. What are you talking about?"

It turns out that one of Olivier's colleagues in a social group approached him to say he had read *Bitter Medicine: A Graphic Memoir of Mental Illness*, the book that Liv and I had created together, in which I had written the text and he had crafted the illustrations. Liv's colleague took exception to Olivier's aspirations to be a visual artist, saw this as Olivier trying to set himself apart from his peers, and said dismissively, "You should stop trying to be a millionaire."

My first response is to track the fellow down, and tell him that, from my experience working in the arts, if Liv wanted to be a *millionaire*, he wouldn't be trying to be an *artist*. There aren't an abundance of millionaire artists out there. Of course, I understand that those kinds of comments spring from jealousy. As in any community, support groups have their share of competition, and some of Liv's colleagues, while they are content to see Liv do well, don't necessarily want to see him do *too* well. Unfortunately, small slights can sink deep with Liv. And now that he's living alone, he has time to brood.

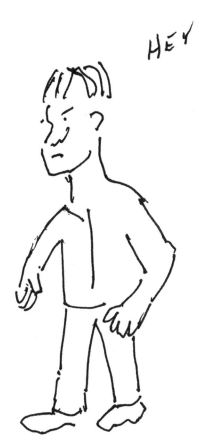

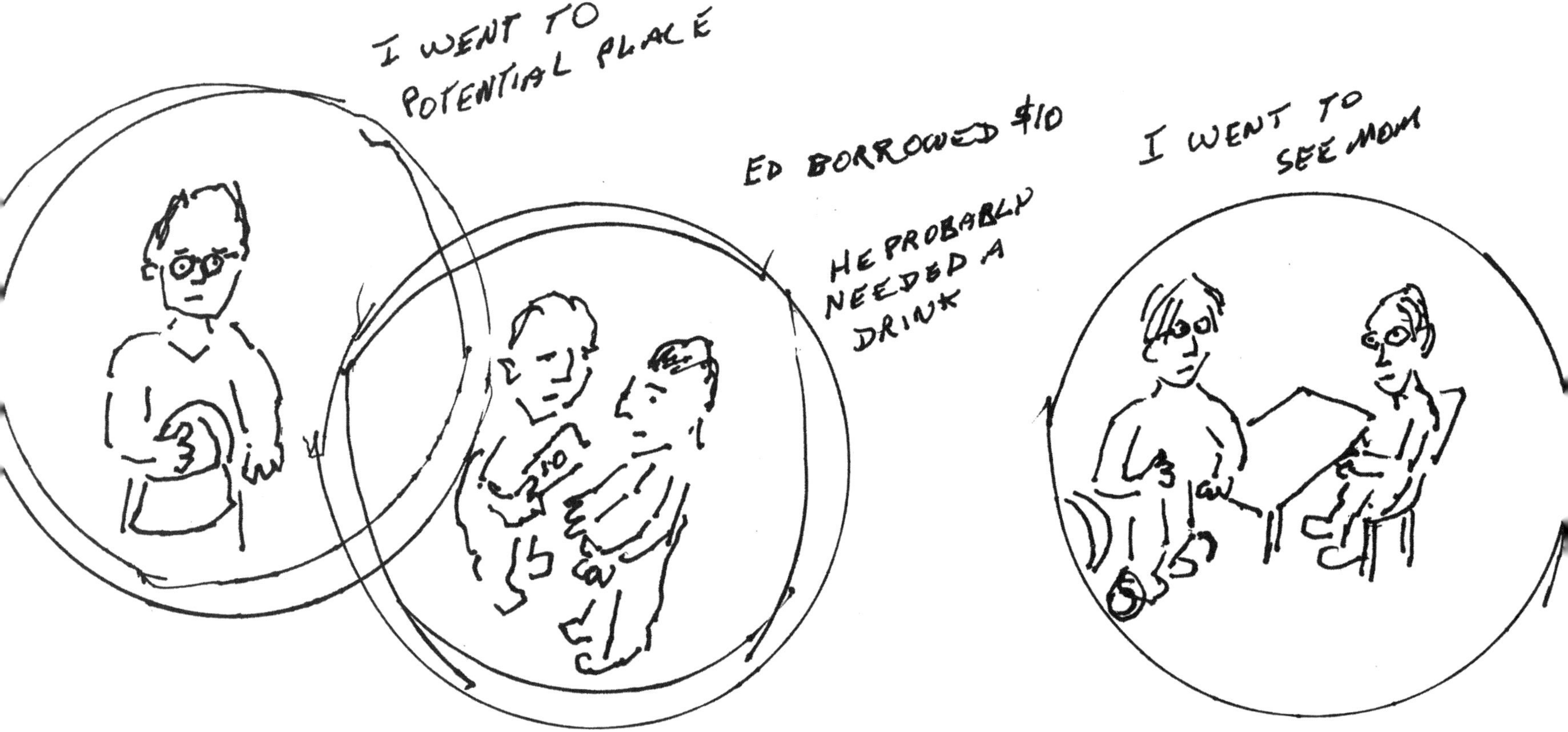
I WENT TO
POTENTIAL PLACE
ED BORROWED $10
HE PROBABLY
NEEDED A
DRINK
I WENT TO
SEE MOM

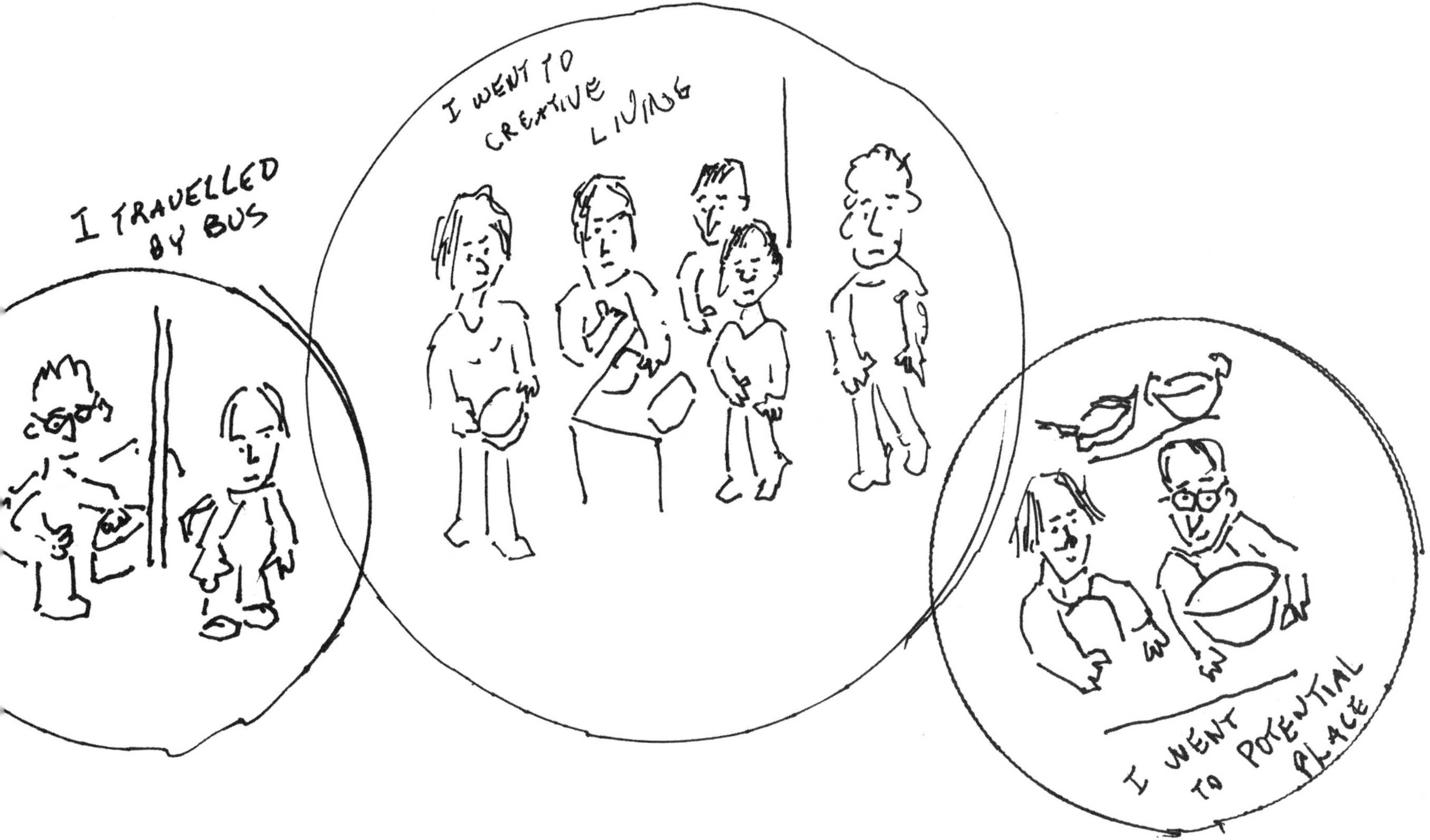
I TRAVELLED BY BUS
I WENT TO CREATIVE LIVING
I WENT TO POTENTIAL PLACE

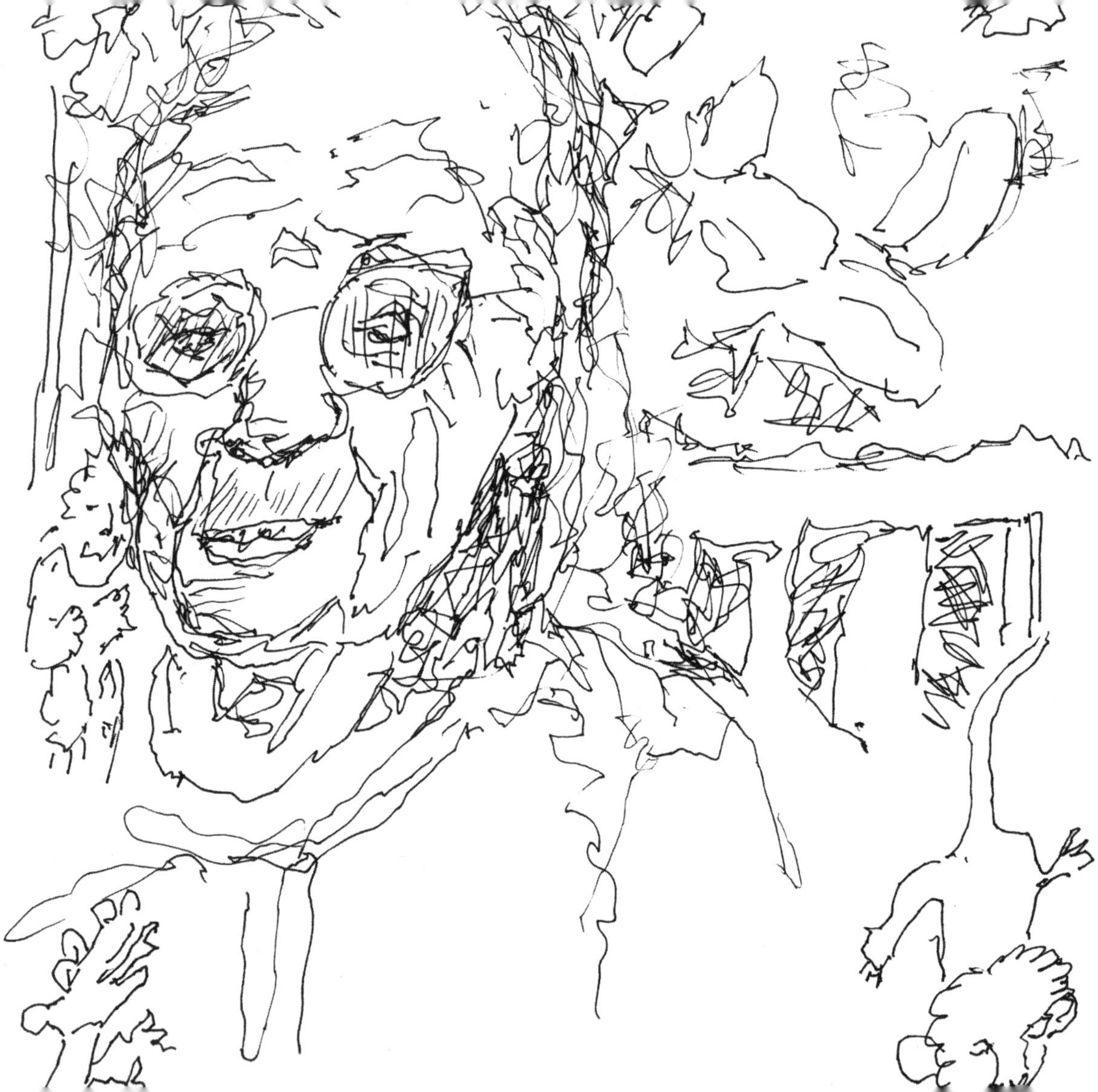

Early in May my mother is finally assessed as requiring long-term care rather than assisted living, which just confirms that our previous search was completely pointless. We scrap our shortlist.

The criteria for the reassessment are, as usual, vague. We're simply informed that our mother is resistant to help, suffers from bowel incontinence, and has mobility and balance issues. All true, of course, but all equally true the first time they assessed her four months ago.

We receive a new list of long-term placements. Summer is approaching, and my mother is now nearing her fourth month in limbo. My brothers and I quickly make our decisions, review the facilities, and create a new shortlist.

Two weeks later I receive a phone call. There's a placement available at the Bow Valley, a facility in the northwest we considered over a year ago. Of all the public facilities, it was our top pick. I drive down to have another look.

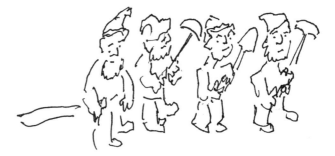

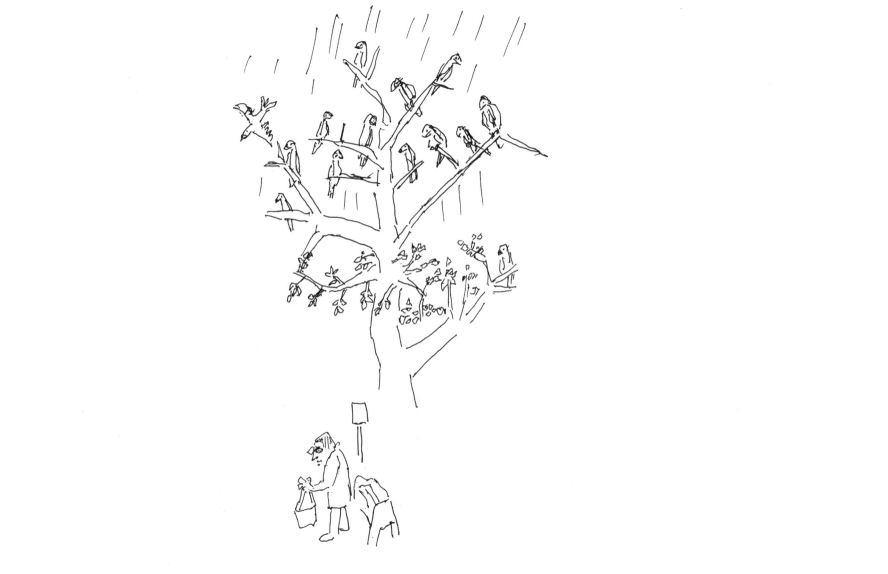

The Bow Valley Long Term Care Facility isn't pretty or modern-looking in the way that the private/public facilities have been, but it has its benefits. It's in a quiet location, close to where Olivier lives so he'll be able to use public transportation. It's one of the smaller facilities, so the staff-to-patient ratio is more manageable. It also has a beautiful central courtyard, a wide open, bright area with skylights two storeys up that permit sunlight to touch all the inward-facing rooms. Trees and plants fill the space, providing a bright, welcoming oasis. I stand in the middle of the courtyard and crane my neck to look up at the light streaming in. Around me, a few clients quietly drink coffee as they assemble puzzles at activity stations.

Maybe this can work.

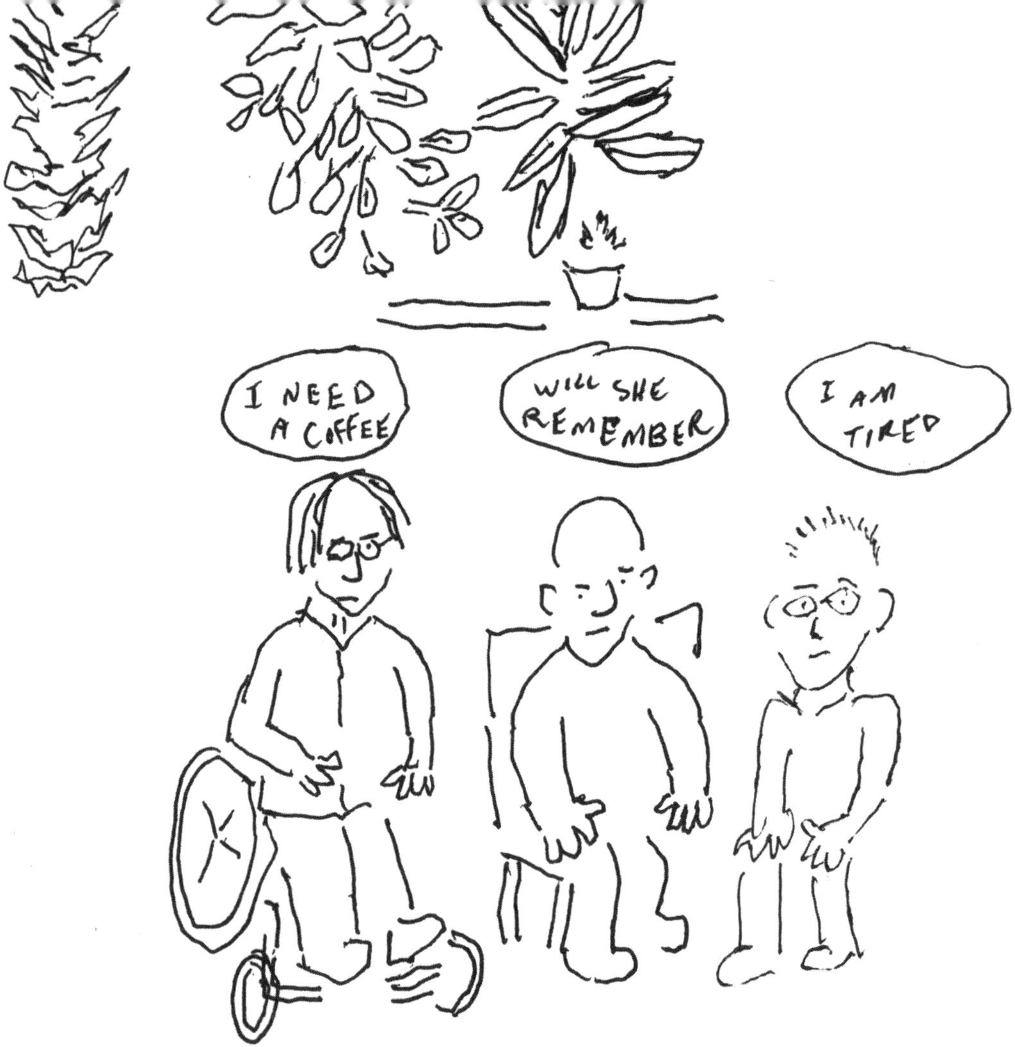
I NEED A COFFEE
WILL SHE REMEMBER
I AM TIRED

I visit Mom to share the news, and find her, as usual, with her hospital gown slipping off one shoulder, crammed behind the door of her room, drinking cold coffee. I offer her water, but she declines. She has suddenly rejected water at the hospital. When I ask why, she raises her eyebrows and asks if I know where they get it. She tells me that she drinks caffeinated coffee instead. I suggest that decaffeinated might be better for her. She frowns and says decaffeinated is for the . . . she searches for the right word and eventually settles on . . . *stupid*.

"Some people feel caffeinated coffee makes them anxious," I observe. She shrugs. "They still worry," she says. "They drink decaffeinated and worry that they won't sleep at night." She takes another sip of her cold coffee. "I drink caffeinated coffee and go right to sleep."

When I tell her she is leaving the hospital tomorrow and transferring to a long-term care facility in her old community, she smiles, finishes her coffee, and murmurs, "Thank heavens."

I hope this will be a good move, but whatever it is, it can't be much of a step down from the transition unit.

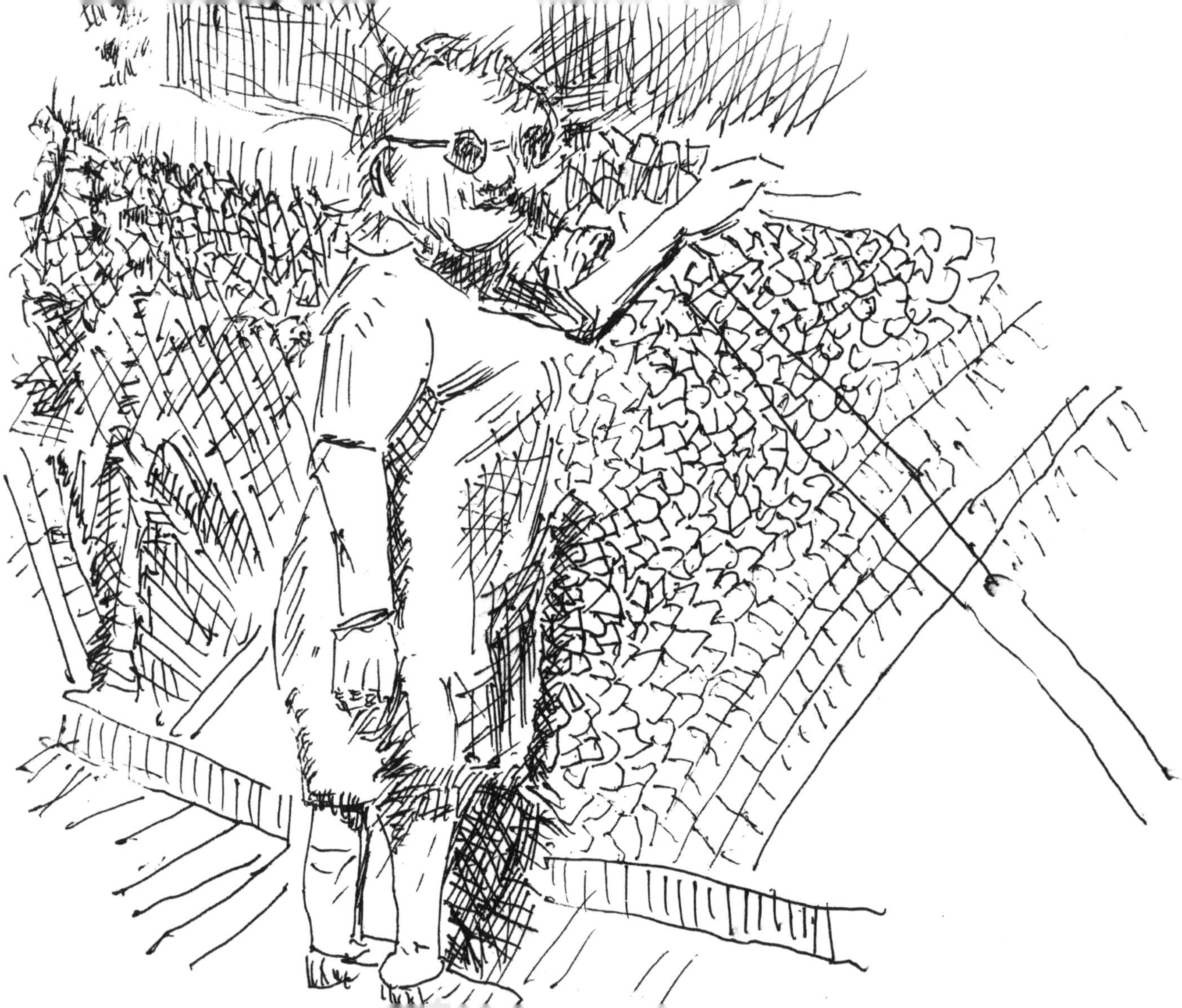

Shortly after breakfast the next day, Mom begins her move. A nurse helps her into a wheelchair and loads her into an ambulance. I assemble her small collection of possessions and drive ahead to meet her.

She will share a bedroom. Her future roommate neither speaks nor moves, and appears unaware of her surroundings. In another time and place, this would be distressing, but in the short term, at least Mom will have little reason to complain about her neighbour talking too much, crying too loudly or stealing — all things she complained about previous roommates.

Her bed and bureau are located next to the courtyard-facing window, offering full access to the natural light of the courtyard's skylights. She likes that. The window opens a crack, allowing air from the garden to circulate. She likes that as well.

While she meets with the physiotherapist — a pleasant, patient woman who appears to be in her last trimester of pregnancy — I slip downstairs to the director's office to fill out forms, organize payments, and set up an incidental account that Mom will be able to draw upon for purchases at the tuck shop or the residents' hair salon.

When I've completed the paperwork, the director takes me to the physiotherapy room, where my mother is arguing with the physiotherapist. Given how unsteady Mom is on her feet and prone to falling, the physiotherapist would prefer that Mom use the wheelchair she was brought in on, but it's a point of pride for my mother that she stand and use her walker, chug along under her own steam. The physiotherapist catches my eye and when I shrug, she acquiesces.

Miriam, an attendant I'd met earlier when I first arrived, peeks in to announce lunch. We exit the physiotherapy room and form a bit of a parade, Miriam leading, my mother following, and me taking up the rear. My mother shoves her walker vigorously ahead of her, defiantly independent, if going at a snail's pace. We eventually enter the dining hall. During her time in the transition unit, Mom has lost weight, so as she walks her pants begin to slither off her hips. Seeing this, Miriam reaches over to tug them up. My mother, surprised at the touch and not understanding that the gesture is intended to help, looks up and glares. Miriam backs off, and I can see that she is appraising my mother, trying to determine just what kind of patient she will be.

Satisfied that she won't be interfered with again, my mother continues lurching across the dining hall floor looking angry and scared. Sixty elderly residents glance up from their meals to watch her.

And suddenly I'm overwhelmed by that feeling you get when you send your child to the first day of school and watch them cross the schoolyard. You know that they're nervous, but you want them to be brave and demonstrate their best behaviour. You want them to be liked and accepted by the others, to find friends and build a community. Only

my mother doesn't smile at anyone, and she doesn't have a neighbourhood chum to accompany her or sit at her table, and this isn't a school or summer camp that she will grow out of or ever leave. This is the final stop.

Fatigued by what for her is a long walk, she wobbles, and another attendant attempts to direct her to her table, but now Mom is anxious, and her temper flares. She snaps at the attendant to keep her hands off. I insert myself to smooth things over, but the attendant gives a quick shake of her head, indicating that it's not necessary for me to say anything, that this kind of response happens all the time. I squeeze in at the table with Mom and two other elderly residents, and talk with her while she eats. Just before I leave she asks me if Clem is going to

come visit. I remind her that I am Clem, and walk away with a knot in my stomach.

Later in the evening, Liv calls and I can hear he's upset. When he visited Mom after dinner she asked if she had to stay at the Bow Valley. He answered yes, that this was where she was living now. She asked him to take her back home. He said he couldn't. She collapsed, crying, saying there was no place for her outside anymore. Liv tells me he wept at the time, and as he recounts the exchange, begins crying again.

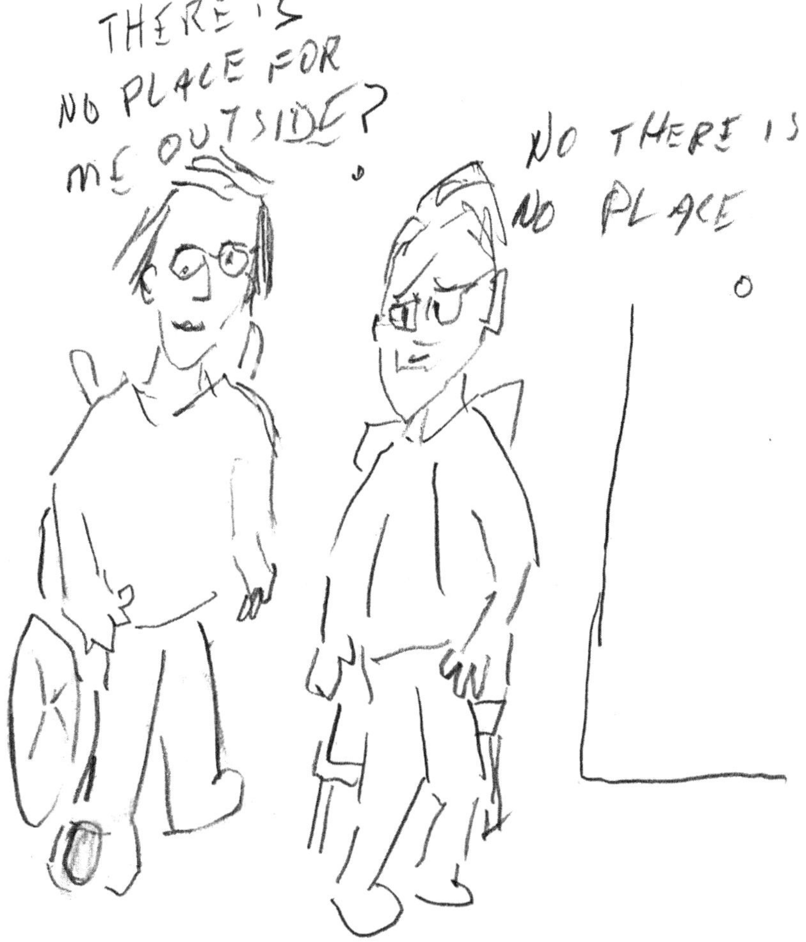
THERE IS
NO PLACE FOR
ME OUTSIDE?
NO THERE IS
NO PLACE

TO DO

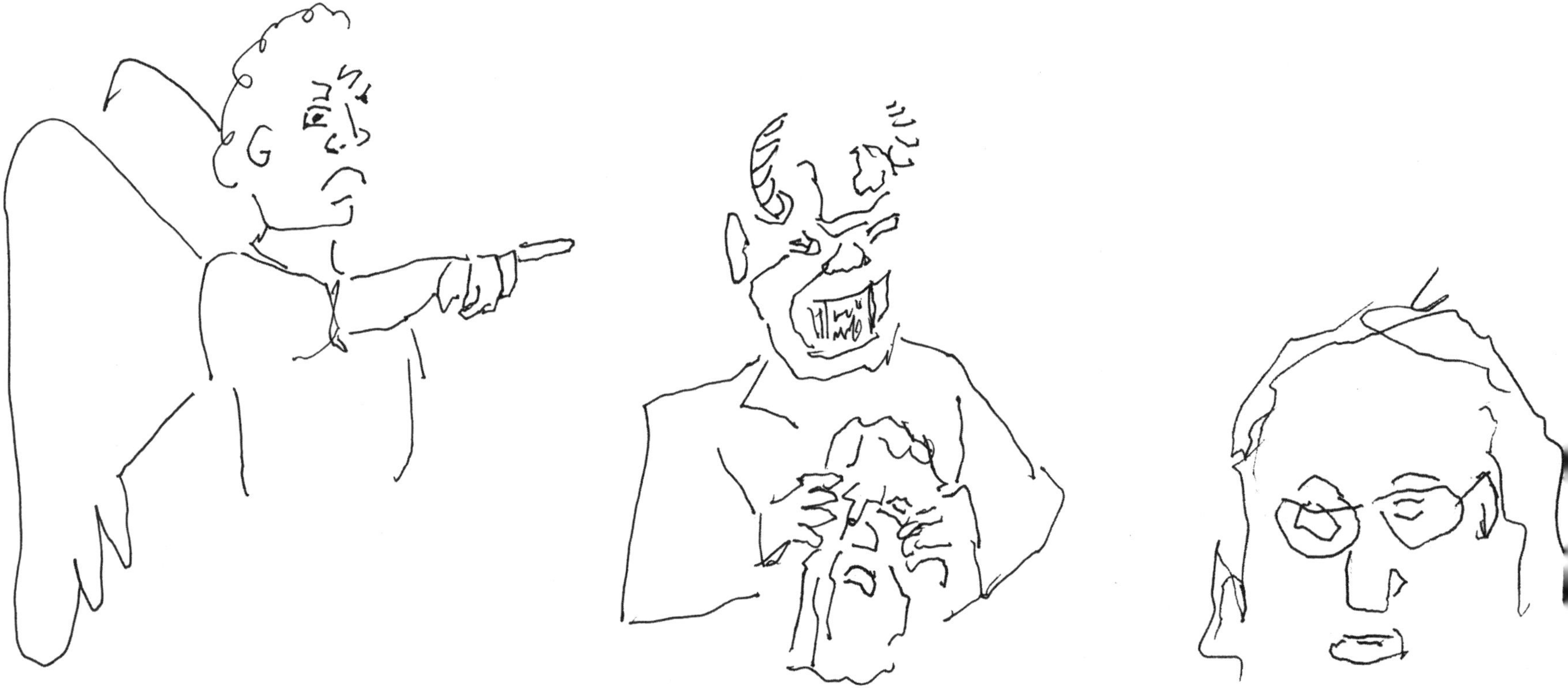

Because my mother is in a long-term care residence, she qualifies through the provincial seniors' benefit for additional funding which, along with her pension and old age security, will cover her room, board, and medical care at the Bow Valley. I put together the application for the benefit, filling out forms and compiling pertinent documents, then mail the package registered post.

Three weeks later, I receive a letter rejecting the application, indicating that an essential form is missing. I check my photocopy of the application. There it is, the duplicate of the form.

I call to correct their mistake, and a machine regretfully informs me that due to a high volume of activity, my wait will be extensive. The voice encourages me to press the number one to leave a message and an employee will return the call at their earliest convenience. I press one, and another machine apologizes and informs me that this mailbox is full, please call again, thanks. Click.

I phone early the next day, hoping to speak to a real person, and go through the same routine. I call at noon, same. No matter when I attempt to speak with someone, early or late, the result is always the same.

In the end, I surrender and simply resubmit everything.

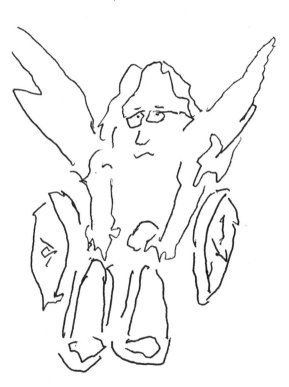

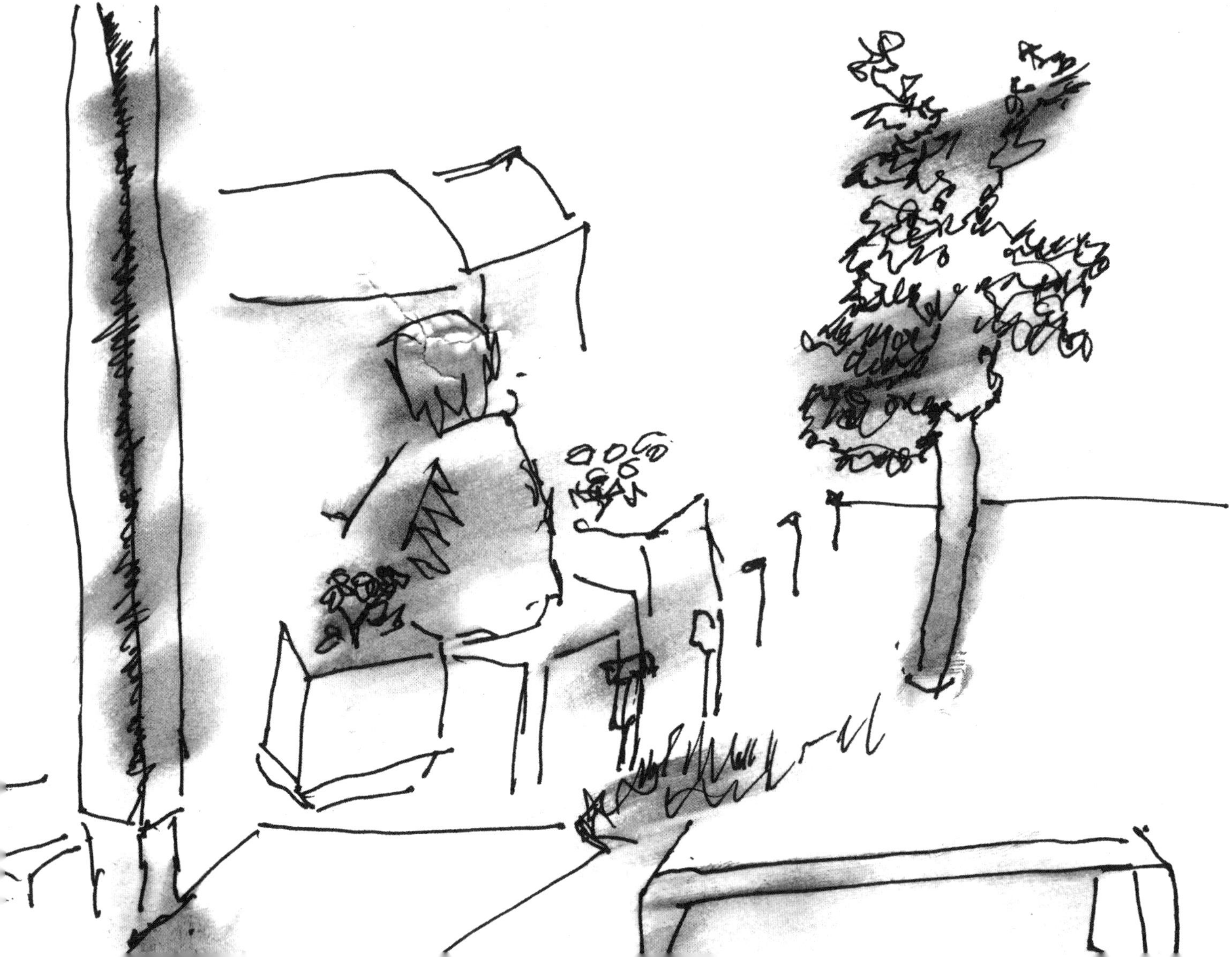

My mother's adjustment to the new facility isn't smooth. During her stay at the transition unit her cognitive abilities continued to decline, and her unwillingness to cooperate hardened into an ingrained instinct. Now she adamantly rejects baths or showers or cleaning of any kind, and the staff have resorted to something like an abduction every couple of days, during which my mother shouts and struggles. The staff approach me to intervene.

I broach the subject with Mom but she remains resolute. She tells me she can feel the water seeping straight through her scalp and skull and into her brain, washing everything away. I suggest that if she wore a shower cap, it might protect her brain. She insists the staff won't permit that, but I assure her they will, and tell her I'll bring a shower cap from home.

Olivier shows up at this point and sits on the bed. I move a jacket aside to make room for him and Mom asks, "Whose jacket is that? Did one of the workers throw it there?"

I glance at the jacket. "It's yours, I think."

"Why would I have a coat out?" she asks.

"Maybe you were cold," I suggest. "You sometimes complain that you get cold, maybe you put it on."

A worker on the other side of the room who is hoisting Mom's roommate into her bed with an electronic lift glances over and says that Mom was wearing the coat earlier. I look closer at the jacket, and read the name tag on it: Catherine Martini.

"It's yours," I confirm, and am thankful that she doesn't pursue it any further.

I've brought cherries to share with Liv and Mom. Mom enjoys them and piles the stones into a little pyramid on a paper napkin while I tell her that at her intake meeting, Karen, the resident social worker, asked us to prepare a life story that we could share with the staff. Something that would allow the workers to know Mom better. What would she like us to tell them?

She says to tell them that a long time ago she grew up in Berlin. After her mother died, she lived alone with her one-armed father. She was conscripted to fight in a war when she was a teenager, and when the war ended and she returned, her father and extended family were all dead. She stops. I wait and when she doesn't continue I tell her that I'll write a draft and have her read and review it.

When Liv and I rise to leave she asks me whose jacket is on her bed. I say it's hers. She tells me to put it away before one of the workers steals it.

I invite Liv over for dinner and take him home following the meal. As soon as we pass through his doorway, he hurries to the washroom and vomits.

When he returns he apologizes and says this often happens. I ask if he's mentioned this to his GP and he grows silent. I imagine he's worried that if he says anything to his doctor, he might be taken off his antipsychotic medication, which he doesn't want to risk. And of course, I don't want to push him to do something he doesn't

want to, but it can't be healthy if he's throwing up after every second meal.

Concerned about his health and frustrated by his unwillingness to deal with it, I glance about the apartment. Dirty socks are strewn in the living room, bags of garbage hedge the door, and dozens of old flyers litter the carpet. I pick up the socks and toss them in a bin by the washing machine, grab a paper towel, and wipe the coffee table down.

The kitchen is awash in stale breadcrumbs, crammed with empty cereal boxes and crusty cans of beans. A cloud of fruit flies swarms me as I scrub the counters. I check the fridge — empty except for an inch of scum-covered brown water and soggy, unidentifiable decomposed fruit in the crisper.

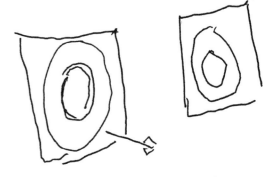

We drain the water and scour the crisper. From now on, I tell Liv, trying to keep my tone even, throw out everything you aren't going to eat, or that looks too old to eat, so it won't attract bugs or mice.

"You're right, Clem," he keeps saying as we wrap the garbage, "you're right."

I feel bossy and controlling and guilty — but the flies and the scummy water . . .

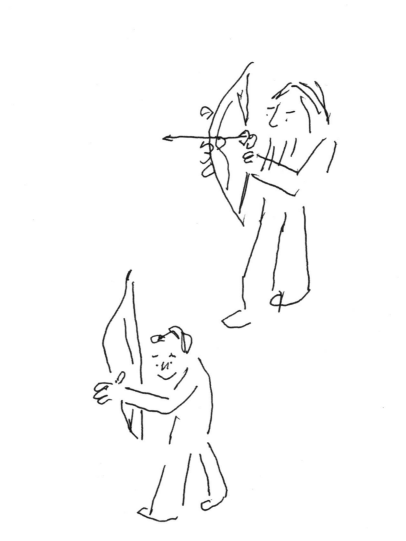

In the early hours of the following day, I lie in the darkness of the bedroom and think about what our family might have been without mental illness or delusions or dementia. How might we have lived our lives had suicide not knocked things over? What might my brothers be doing? Who might we have been?

A current philosophy winding its way through the mental health culture posits, in essence, that since mental illness has always existed and always will exist, it should be accepted. If we can't actually generate a cure, we can at least alter the conditions that stigmatize and "other" those who have it. So, we should make room for it. Embrace it. "Make friends with it," one person suggested to me.

And, of course, every effort should be made to eliminate the stigma associated with mental illness — there's no excuse for discrimination or exclusion — but on the other hand, I hate that kind of slack, shallow, sage-sounding advice. Certainly, I'll live with schizophrenia, and my brother will live with schizophrenia, we'll all live with it — what choice have we got? But as for being friends with it? Frankly I say screw making nice with schizophrenia. I am angry at schizophrenia. I am furious at the pain and damage it causes. I don't want to "embrace" schizophrenia — a disorder that killed one brother and torments another — I want to see it cured. I want to see the same kind of energy and commitment and passion and financial resources that are presently devoted to finding a cure for heart disease, for MS, for cancer — that are devoted to finding a cure for premature hair loss, for goodness sake — devoted to ending schizophrenia.

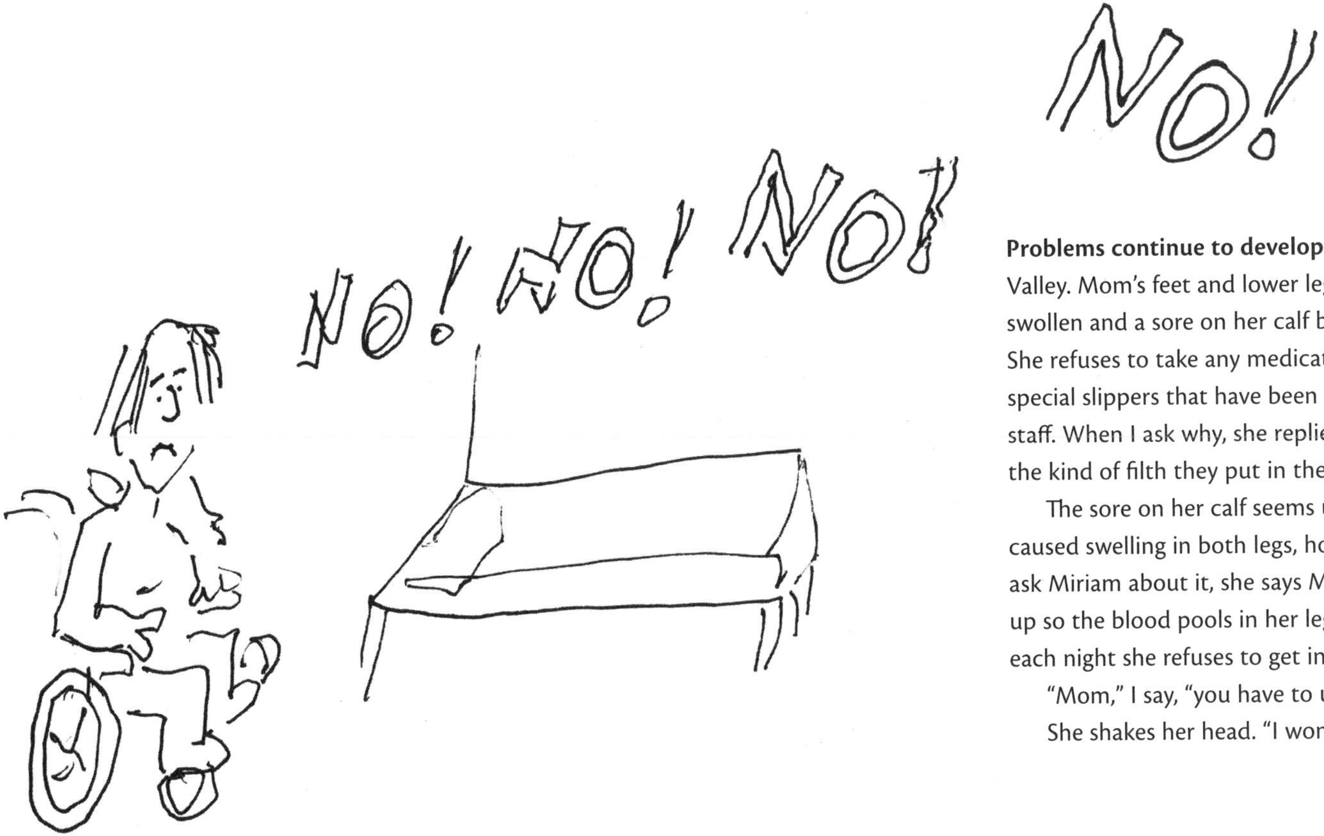

NO! NO! NO! NO!

Problems continue to develop at the Bow Valley. Mom's feet and lower legs have become swollen and a sore on her calf becomes infected. She refuses to take any medication or wear the special slippers that have been provided by the staff. When I ask why, she replies, "Do you know the kind of filth they put in there?"

The sore on her calf seems unlikely to have caused swelling in both legs, however. When I ask Miriam about it, she says Mom sleeps sitting up so the blood pools in her legs. Apparently each night she refuses to get into her bed.

"Mom," I say, "you have to use your bed."

She shakes her head. "I won't."

"Why not?" I ask. "You slept in your bed at home."

"I'm not lying in bed with every Tom, Dick, and Harry," she says.

That catches me by surprise. "I'm pretty certain," I assure her, "that your bed is empty and ready for you each night."

"No," she insists. "There's someone under the covers every night, and I won't sleep with them!"

I don't know how to argue with that. I'm out of my depth. On my way out, I tell the staff what she told me, and they say they'll try giving the bed a quick sweep with a hand at bedtime to prove that no one is lying there.

I find it so strange that my mother, who was once fearless about spending the night in a sleeping bag in the wilderness in the worst kind of weather, now refuses to lie in her bed. These kinds of changes make me question everything I thought I knew about identify. You love someone, think you know them, then one day that someone changes. Who has she become? The person you knew liked to drink water, now she doesn't. The person you knew used to complete crossword puzzles every evening, now she doesn't know what to do with one. The person you loved was competent and tidy and organized. No longer. With each passing month, week, even day, another aspect of the original person is pared away, leaving only shreds and fragments and splinters.

My mother also struggles to cling to her memories of me, to recall who I am, to recollect experiences we've shared. On good days memories flood back, but increasingly I am just another vaguely remembered relative. A son, usually — but one of three or four?

And that erasure of memory tests everything. To a degree, the person you love is always a constructed memory, or a compilation of memories, some distant, some recent. I love my mother because of all the moments we've shared, the care she's shown for me, the sacrifices she made on my behalf. What happens if her memories of these shared events are lost? What if my memories of these things are vandalized by this disorder — who will I love then? And because my own identity is formed in relation to all of my shared experiences, who will I become?

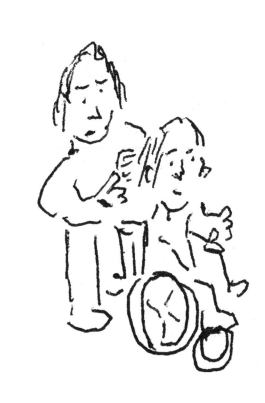

A PEST
ON YOU!

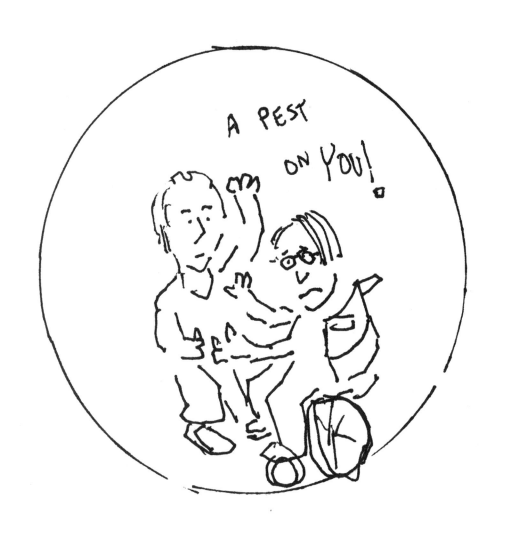

The Bow Valley goes on lockdown because of an outbreak of viral gastroenteritis. Residents who have contracted the virus are confined to their bedrooms, second-floor residents (my mother among them) are not permitted to travel to the first floor, and visitors are not permitted to travel between floors. After several days of this, things break down under the strain. One elderly woman sings a mournful song loudly and off-key in the hallway. Another cries that she wants to go out, she wants to go out! Another follows me into my mom's room, stands staring at us, and refuses to leave. A nurse enters moments later and guides her out.

My mother becomes confused and alarmed by the orange strips of tape that bar entry into rooms designated as quarantined. Unable to visit the courtyard — the venue we generally migrate to for coffee — I instead take her to the TV room. The television is turned to mute, and the images scroll silently as my mother concentrates on slowly peeling a banana. She snaps off an end portion, chews it for some time, then sets the rest aside. She closes her eyes and breathes deeply. I ask if she is all right. She doesn't answer.

Abruptly she announces in a loud voice her urgent need to use the washroom. I have her place her feet back on the wheelchair's foot supports, and push her in the direction of her room. Along the way, I ask one of the attendants to give my mother a hand. They slip into the washroom together. Minutes pass and the attendant returns, her face flushed, to ask if I will help. Mom is being uncooperative.

When I step into the tiny washroom I am confronted by something that looks more like a street fight than a medical intervention. My mother is facing down three attendants, furiously batting away their hands. They're trying to strap a belt around her waist to lift her, and she can't figure out what's going on.

"Just help me up," she shouts. I tell her that that is what they are trying to do, but she can't hear me — there's too much noise in that small space, and of course she's hollering at the same time. The nurses are shouting as well, shouting at her and calling directions to one another.

"Lean in, take her *under the arms!*"

"I'm trying to secure *the strap!*"

My mother darts a panicked glance at me. "Look," she says, "there are three of them and only one of me!" as though she's preparing to take them on, and needs me by her side to even the odds.

I lean in to help lift her, but the whole operation is in flux now. Five of us are crammed into a room meant to accommodate one and my mother keeps shrieking and slapping away hands, like it is the fight of her life. In the end the senior nurse raises her voice above the din and orders all the other assistants to vacate the room. She and I stay behind. Mom briefly stops struggling, panting as she tries to recover. The nurse directs me to lift Mom by the waist strap now that it's been secured. It's difficult, because although Mom isn't heavy, until she places her feet firmly beneath her there's a risk that she'll take a tumble. Slowly Mom inches

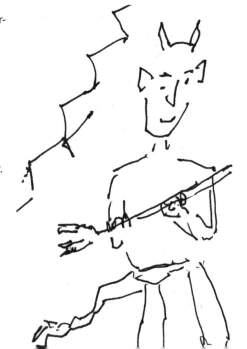

to the edge of the wheelchair, plants her hands on the arms of the chair, and strains to push off. The nurse and I grab the lifting belt and heave. I hold Mom there, mid-air, as she once more screams, frightened that she can neither really stand nor sit. With one foot, I kick the wheelchair out of the way. As Mom dangles by the waist strap, the senior nurse directs her to adjust her legs and walk back toward the toilet. My mother moves one foot. I urge her to keep going. Together, we slowly lower her onto the toilet seat. It is a protracted, strenuous, surreal process, but finally successful.

When it's finished, I am soaked through with sweat. I stand, straighten my back, and think, "Surely, *surely* it can't be this way every time she has to use the washroom."

I leave the room feeling sorry for my mother — what a graceless, humiliating, invasive exercise. I feel sorry for the attendants as well — it's the very definition of a thankless job, trying to help someone who is resisting help with all her might. And I feel a little sorry for myself.

As I wait in the hallway, a nurse informs me that my mother has been holding back her bowel movements. I can see why, if going to the toilet causes this kind of commotion each time. Twenty minutes later my mother still hasn't emerged. I'm late to attend a meeting, so I shout goodbye through the washroom door. I'm not sure she hears.

It's as if age is a fire that Mom is slowly being lowered into, and it burns away everything that existed but her essence. My mother's independent spirit, always so important to her, remains, but it's twisted into an almost unrecognizable shape by the intense heat. Instead of being helpful to her, this disfigured, charred independence compels her to refuse help. It makes her most miserable in her time of misery, most alone in a time when she could use a friend, most unable to differentiate between foes and allies.

What has happened to her kindness, her intelligence, her sense of humour, her dignity? All consumed in the flames. And I cannot help but feel that as I approach the heat I am scorched as well. I feel a tightness of flesh, a congealing. I feel hardened, as though all the liquids that kept me supple and resilient have been boiled away.

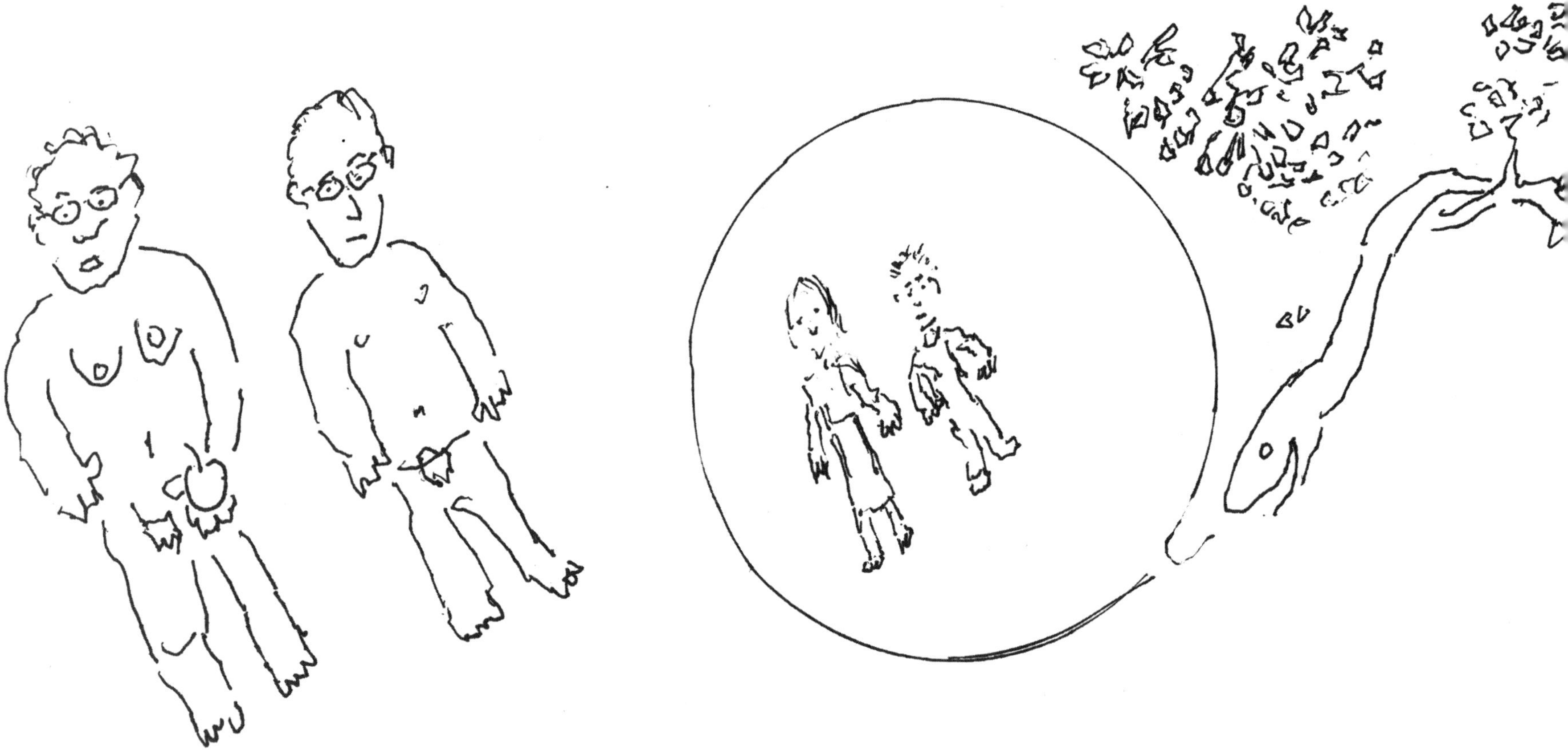

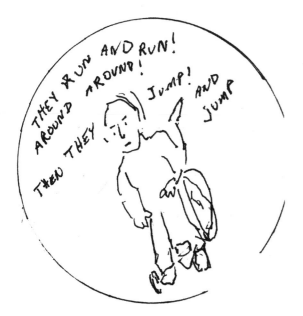

THEY RUN AND RUN!
AROUND AROUND!
THEN THEY JUMP! AND JUMP

A bruise emerges on Mom's wrist the following day, and a long red welt beneath her chin. A few days later another purple discoloration appears above her right cheek. My mother explains that these were put there by a "hated nurse." That the staff treat her worse than a prisoner, and do anything they want to her. I object that they seem nice enough when I'm there. She tells me she didn't sleep in the bed last night because the nurses placed ice on one side of her, and then ice on the other side, and then pulled an enormous sheet of ice over top of her to immobilize her and keep her quiet.

I'm not sure what to make of the sheet of ice, but even though I can imagine that she could have hit her wrist, chin, and cheek against the railing in her flailing about the other day, I worry about the bruises. I've read stories of elder abuse and it's not hard to imagine someone losing their temper when my mother is incensed.

But how do you advocate on behalf of someone whose perception is so skewed that she believes attendants are encasing her in ice? And how can I determine which concerns are valid, when so many are imagined? I raise the matter of the bruises and the ice with staff, who maintain that the injuries are all self-generated, and that there have been no sheets of ice. That's as far as it goes, but at least there's a record of my concerns, and I have a note to reference if other bruises appear in the future.

And then only days later I'm sitting at home watching the news when the announcer warns that the following video contains graphic footage that may prove disturbing. She's right.

Three attendants at another long-term care facility across town have been arrested, tried, and imprisoned for abusing an elderly client. The man, bedridden, stiff with age and suffering from advanced prostate cancer, complained to his family that he was afraid of his nurses. The family planted a hidden camera in his room. Footage of the abuse was submitted as evidence at the trial and a clip is now shown on the news. It's horrific. Three middle-aged women roughly change the old man, picking him up and tossing him down on the bed,

splashing urine in his face. They punch and slap him, drag the bedsheets over his head and press down, smothering him. They dart in to poke him, and the obvious relish they take from outraging and abusing the old man is obscene. It feels like an image pulled from some dark and arcane medieval woodcut of a Black Sabbath. It's so violent, so calculated to demean and humiliate, that it is absolutely chilling, and at the same time it is so clearly arising out of feelings of powerlessness and repressed frustration.

The elderly are hidden away in these institutions and are, for many, many hours, totally at the mercy of their caregivers. The residents' lack of coherence, of cognition, of memory, render them entirely and tragically vulnerable.

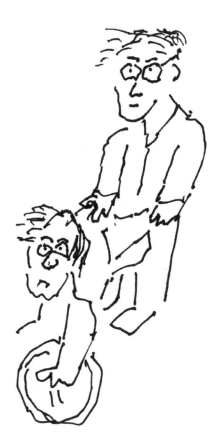

Staff, on the other hand, are so poorly paid, and so transient from one institution to another, that it makes good people difficult to find, adequate supervision almost impossible, and criminal incidents such as the one described almost inevitable.

Of course I have no indication that anything like this is occurring with my mother — the staff seem kind and tolerant — but short of secretly installing my own video camera, how would I know for sure? The images stay with me for a long time after I've turned the television off.

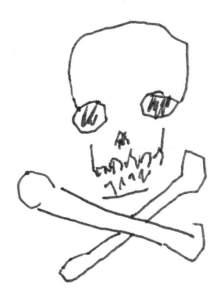

A few days later I call Liv when I know he'll have returned from his support group, just to see how he's doing. He sounds sad and says he's had a tough day. He thinks one of his group members, a fellow he's had trouble with before, is planning to do something bad. He says he heard this fellow say, "We'll see how smart he feels after we take care of him."

When I ask what he believes this fellow's intentions are, he reveals a long plot that involves setting Liv up in some incriminating context, then photographing him, then extorting funds from him.

I listen for a while, then say, "Liv, did you actually hear any of this?"

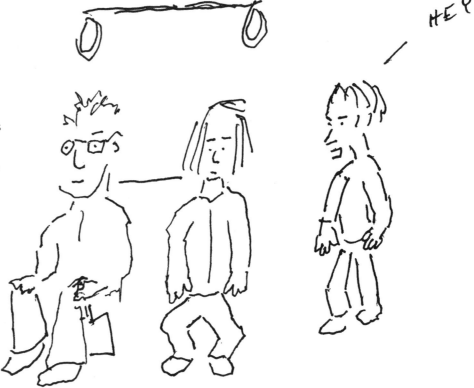

He considers the question a long moment, then says, "No."

"So this is something you thought up?"

"Not thought up, exactly."

I confront once more the imprecise terminology that exists for describing a delusion. "But you didn't actually hear it?" I ask.

"No."

I suggest that he avoid hanging out with the fellow for a while, and that he bring up these feelings with his psychiatrist when they next meet.

He thanks me and we talk a few more moments, then say good night. When I hang up, I continue chewing on the conversation.

Here's the difficulty — there are a number of ways of viewing the conversation, and which is correct?

Maybe it's real, all of it. There are, after all, real, actual criminals in the world, and there are some genuinely rough characters who attend Liv's support groups, some who have had their run-ins with the law and spent time behind bars. Maybe there is someone who holds a grudge against Liv and maybe he actually does intend to act on that grudge. Then again, maybe Liv's description is only partially based on the circumstances. It could be that there's someone in his group who has had an issue with Liv in the past, but Liv has misjudged the scale of the grudge and capability of the individual. Or maybe it's all delusion and paranoia.

So when Olivier says, as he does just before we finish our conversation, "If you find me beaten to death, you will know that it was Greg," I'm left asking, how should I respond?

Should I take it as a criminal matter — contact the police and have Greg investigated? Should I take it as a medical matter — that is, determine if Liv needs to adjust his medication or get additional psychiatric attention? Or should I just take it under advisement, and wait to see how things develop?

At this point, I lean toward the latter two, but what if I'm wrong? What if I wake one day to find that he has, in fact, been beaten to death?

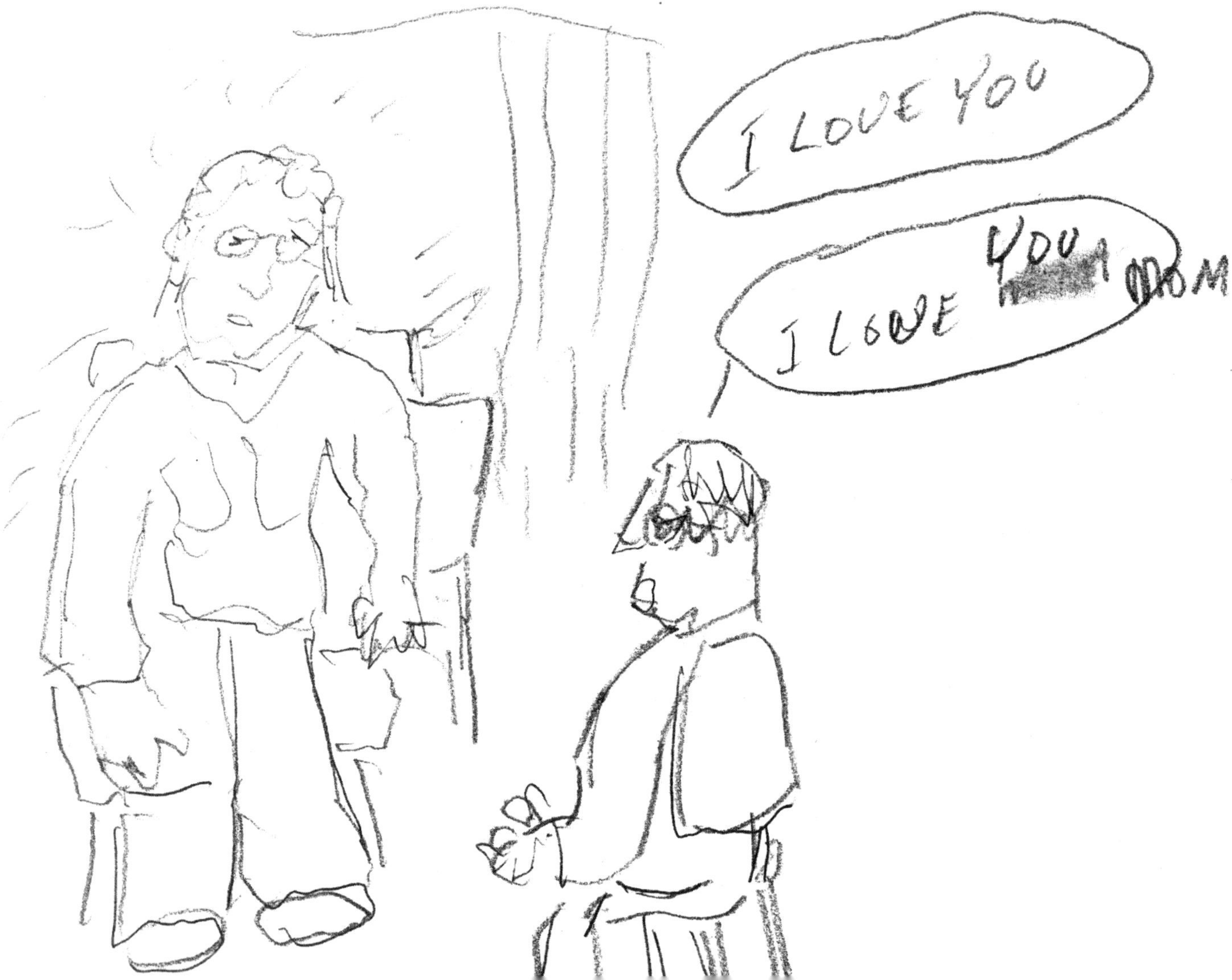
I LOVE YOU
I LOVE YOU MOM

Some time ago I brought two shower caps for Mom and requested that staff use them during her showers. I notice that one is missing, and ask Mom whether she tried it. She says she did, but then the care workers removed it and "scrubbed and scrubbed and scrubbed" until water was forced into her brain.

Even touching on the issue of showers is a delicate matter, and once the topic is broached my mother's anger mounts. I try changing the subject but she won't be distracted. She tells me that being at the Bow Valley is like serving time in prison, that the attendants act like guards, that she wishes she was dead, *dead*, and says I wouldn't care if she were.

"The only one that loves me is Olivier," she rails, "and you've never cared for him!"

"That's not true," I reply.

Her shouts are attracting the attention of the others in the courtyard. "You forgot all about him and if the Unitarian Church hadn't helped him—"

"The Unitarian Church didn't do anything for him—"

"—he would have been shoved out."

"Shoved him out of *where*?" I demand, my heart racing and my voice rising in turn. "What are you talking about? Your involvement with the Unitarian Church was beside the point. That the Unitarian Church did anything regarding Liv's schizophrenia is just another of your delusions."

"Oh yes! That's right," she spits, nodding her head up and down as though confirming a long-held suspicion. "You just think I'm nuts!"

"Okay, look," I snap, pushing myself out of the chair. "I've got to go."

I unlock the wheelchair, seize the handles, and move toward the elevator. As I take her up to her bedroom, we're angry and silent, and I realize even as I park her back in her bedroom that I shouldn't have participated in the argument. What use was there in listening to her accusations, or shouting, or bickering with her? What use was any of it?

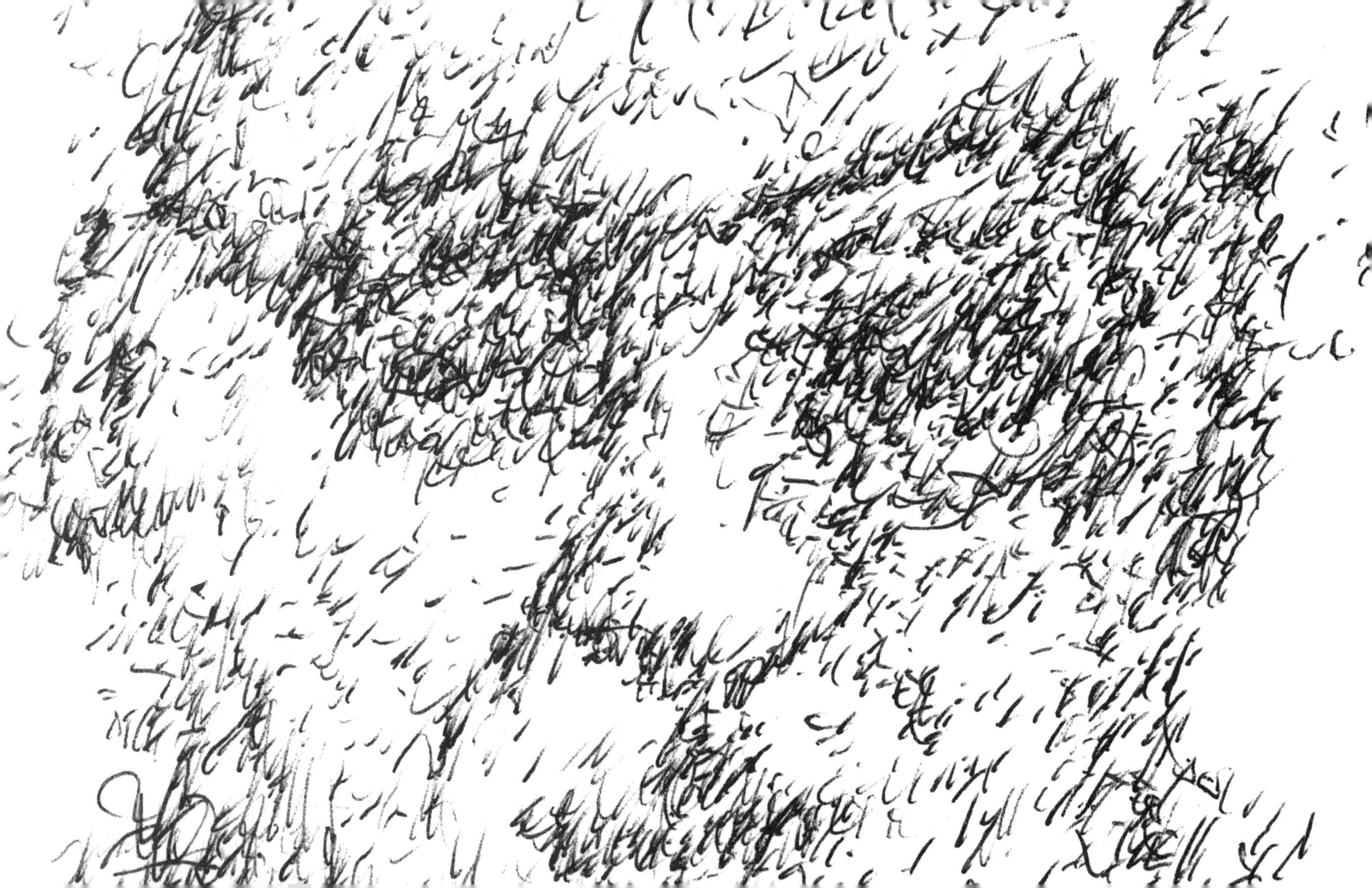

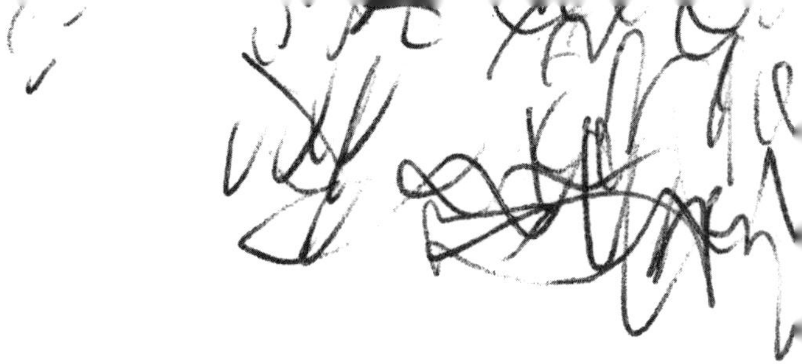

At my annual physical I sit on the examination table and as my doctor's checking my reflexes, she asks how I am doing. When I tell her my sleep is troubled, she glances up at me. What do I mean by troubled? I wake early and lie sleepless in the dark, I say, then feel exhausted the next day.

She asks what's going on in my life, and when I tell her, she says, "That sounds difficult." True, I think, but unremarkable. From my observations, everybody's life is difficult.

She runs through the basics of something she calls "sleep hygiene": keep regular hours, minimize caffeine intake, clear the bedroom of TVs, computers and other distractions. Then she suggests an exercise that might help. When I am lying awake at night I should imagine three different sensory objects. Something I can touch. Something I can smell. Something I can taste. The mind, she assures me, cannot maintain anxiety and three separate sensory items all at once. Or alternately, she says, she can provide me with prescription drugs. I appreciate her concern, but don't want any medication, and tell her that won't be necessary.

I try to follow the doctor's advice, but my anxiety appears able to thrive regardless of how many sensory objects I apply. It clings to me regardless of where I am or what I am doing. It seeps deep inside and stains everything: my work, my home, my family.

The day following my visit with the doctor, while seated at my desk at work, I decide to call a counsellor on the help line provided by the university. In days past I would have made my way to a stuffy office, taken a comfortable, worn seat, spoken with someone face to face. Now counselling is outsourced to a private corporation, and the service is provided at a distance over the phone.

I dial in, and an electronic voice reminds me that everything we say will be recorded. Seconds later, Anna, my counsellor for this session, is on the line, asking me what I am feeling. Stretched thin, I say. I feel like a failure. I don't know what I'm doing and I am over-whelmed. I feel like I have taken on tasks that are beyond me, bigger than me, and that they never get easier and they never get smaller. Anna murmurs encouragingly, sometimes repeating what I have said for clarification, sometimes probing. Am I losing weight, she asks? Do I suffer from fatigue? Have I concerns that I will do self-harm? I say no, but even as I answer her, a paralyzing feeling of uselessness envelops me. What can she do from her telephone miles away — or if she were sitting right in front of me, for that matter? How can she change the facts? The facts are inescapable. My brother struggles with a disease that daily threatens to overpower him, and none of my efforts can eradicate it. My mother is dying incrementally, one brain cell at a time. Nothing can change that. I can't create a situation that will make her happy or give her peace.

Through the chatter of my own thoughts, I hear the counsellor continue speaking to me.

"Pardon me?" I ask.

"What do you want to achieve?" she repeats. "Do you want actions that will change your situation or do you want to find ways to feel better about the present situation?"

I want to be able to breathe again.

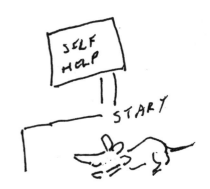

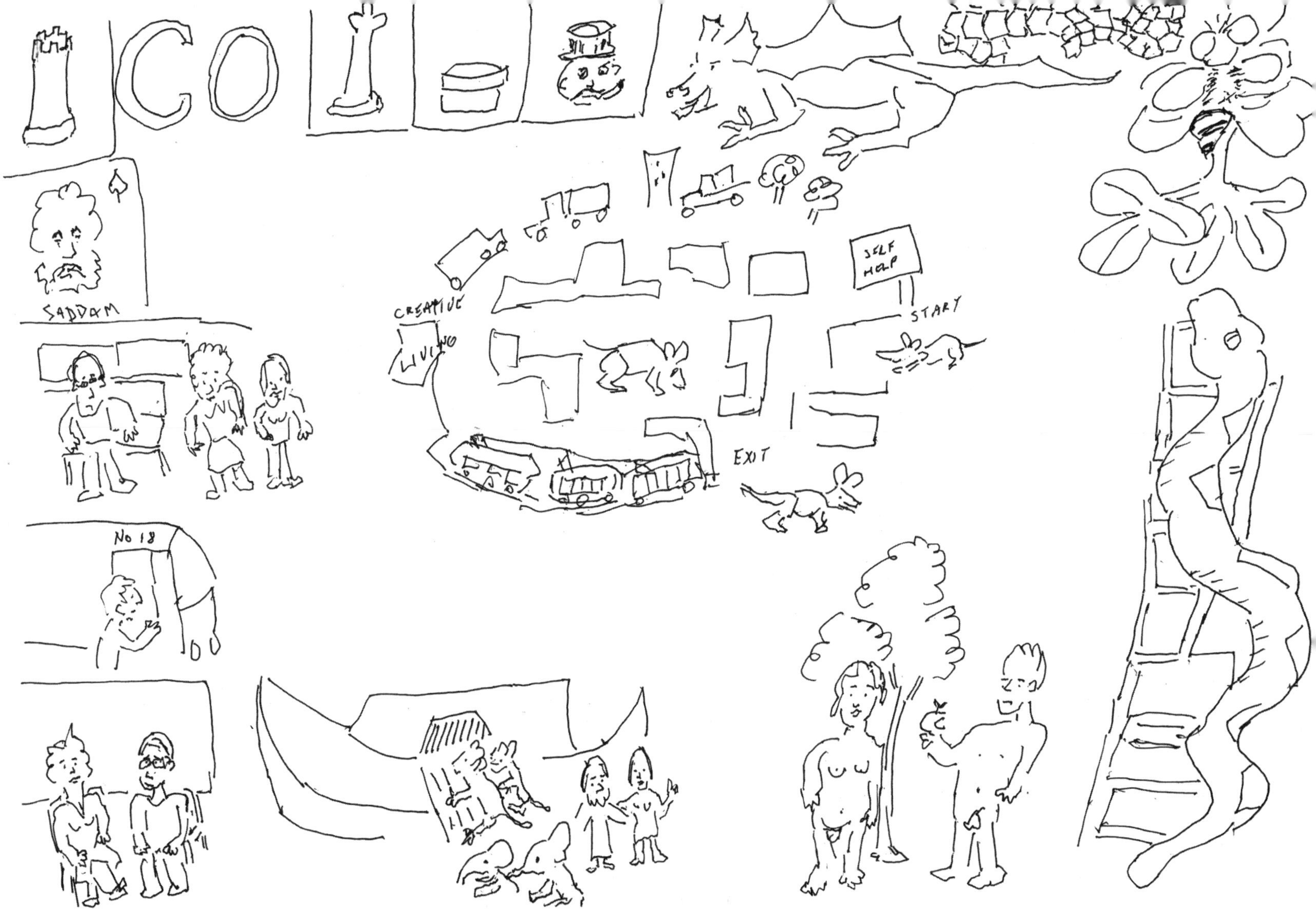

SADDAM
CREATIVE
LIVING
SELF HELP
START
EXIT
No 18

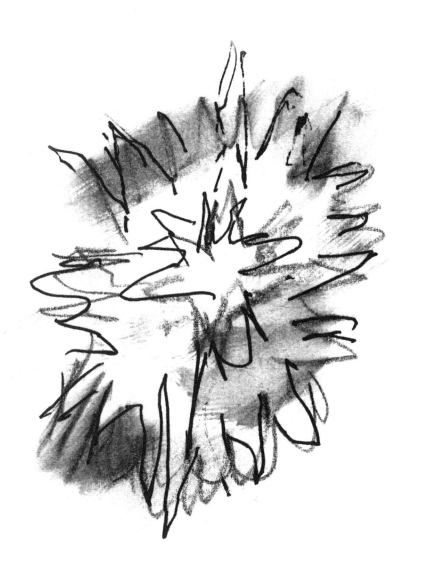

The migraine appears unbidden in a sudden glittering slash of zigzagging light on the left side of my brain, solidifies into a tender throbbing vein in my temple that radiates pain through my entire skull.

It's the long weekend. Nic is out of town with his family in Waterton, and Olivier is attending a retreat at Camp Goldeye with his supportive living group, so Mom won't get any visitors if I don't go. As I drive to the Bow Valley, the world billows and rocks, sound is louder and harsher than usual, light is brighter. When I enter Mom's bedroom, she's seated in her wheelchair, facing her desk. Her hair is matted and a brown stain trails down her chin and onto her shirt. I pluck a Kleenex from a box, wipe her chin, and offer to take her downstairs for coffee. As we vacate her room, a care worker sidles alongside, whispering that Mom needs a shower and asking me to help persuade her. I mumble that I'll try.

My head pounds. My mother and I find seats in the courtyard and talk generally for a few moments about the weekend and my kids. I tentatively raise the matter of showering and she instantly transitions to full-on fury.

"They are pouring water all over me!" she shrieks, loudly enough that a lady across the courtyard giving her mother a manicure looks up, concerned. "All over me! Pouring water over my face, over my face and into my brain!"

Her voice is piercing. I have run out of ideas. There's nothing left. I give up. I wheel her back to her room and leave her for someone else to take to dinner.

The next day, once I'd recovered from my migraine, I return to try once more to convince my mother to take a shower. That won't be necessary, she tells me, all she needs is her special hairbrush. This hairbrush, she says, and a hundred strokes will clean her hair — and by extension, I suppose, her. I express my concern that this won't pass muster with the staff. "Nothing," she says, tossing the hairbrush aside, "I do is right."

Meant as a statement of defiance, it is at the same time a forlorn surrender, a recognition that she no longer holds the power to make decisions that others view as good ones, and it evokes in me feelings of intense frustration, genuine pity — and familiarity.

Nothing I do is right. I feel that as well. My frustration bleeds into my work. Frustration with colleagues in the workplace who refuse to speak with one another, who decline to sit on committees, who bicker over the minutest points of difference. Frustration at the seemingly endless cost-cutting "exercises" that my workplace administration directs us to embark on. At another time I might have had patience for these things, but now I have none. I feel squeezed into a corner. Every troubled event collects on top of me, like particles of dust settling in an ancient library until the bookcases bow and shatter under the accumulated weight. I lie awake nights with these thoughts turning and turning about.

When I get home, I tell Cher that I think I may need a retreat. That's what I'm calling it. A retreat. That sounds better than "an escape." She asks if there's anything she can do.

I say no, that I'm just going to go to Cypress Hills Provincial Park to clear my head. When we rise in the morning, we have tea, and I pack my things. She hands me a lunch she's put together, gives me a hug, and asks me to call when I arrive at the campsite to let her know I'm all right.

I throw my backpack and tent in the trunk of the car, climb behind the wheel, and set out. I drive six hours south, through a long, flat, dry pan of prairie. The horizontal line is immense — a broad flat, uniformly gold and tan stretch of grass and short brush, like an enormous piece of toffee stretched into the thinnest membrane. Then suddenly, the landscape tilts and I'm gliding down an incline dipping south and east into the Mississippi River Basin. I turn off the highway just after Medicine Hat, winding and swooping through rolling hills into Cypress Hills Provincial Park. Trees edge the gullies and gorges, and tall grasses sway along the crests of hills.

At Spruce Coulee campsite, I park, then hoist and carry my backpack to an empty site, toss the rolled up tent to the earth. The place looks near deserted. Only three other campers have claimed places. The air is thick with the scent of pine. I unbag the tent, slip poles through it, raise it, and fasten it tight with pegs, then zip it open and toss in my sleeping bag.

A squirrel peers at me, then springs acrobatically from the grass to a tree trunk and quickly shimmies into the canopy. Restless, I set out walking along a portion of the Trans Canada Trail, an imposing track that stretches east to the Atlantic Coast and west to the Pacific, but here is just an unassuming dirt path edged by sedges and wild rose bushes. The trail slips through groves of aspen and alder, the wind sweeps over me, and I hope it will scour me of my unease.

I walk and walk and encounter no one. The soft earth gives under my feet; the musky scent of dust and sage rises with every step. I try to still the clatter in my brain, limit my thoughts to what I see and hear and touch. The wind rifles the grass tops. A barn owl floats across a field, enormous feathery wings and silence. A moose stalks through tall reeds and turns its broad, impossibly long head to gaze at me with strangely deep and peaceful eyes. At dusk, I return to camp. It's quiet and still, the only sound the chatter of wind in the upper boughs of the poplars.

Night drops and I build a campfire. I grill sausages and potatoes, open a can of beans, and brew tea. I scrape the sausage, potatoes, and beans onto a dish, eat them hot, then rinse the plates under the pump and leave them to dry in a rack. Stretching out atop the rough wooden picnic table, I gaze up at the sky. It is like peering down the darkest mouth of the largest, deepest well.

I stay awake late, poking the embers and avoiding sleep. The wonderful thing, though, about overnighting in the tent is that the cold is so biting and the ground so uncomfortable that it allays my fears of being tormented by dreams. My hip becomes acquainted with a lumpy root I hadn't detected when I erected the tent; the nape of my neck is introduced to a projecting rock. Finally, in the early morning,

I manage to drowse, and while I hover between sleep and wakefulness, my mother visits me. She sits in her wheelchair, slowly turns, looks at me, and says, "Nothing I do is right."

I wake to mist clinging to the trees, and a different kind of silence, thick and cottony. The sun emerges a pale disc, casting no more heat than it does light. I throw together a quick breakfast of granola and milk, then clean up and spend the rest of the day hiking, mostly on my own, although at one bend in the trail I encounter a father with his two small sons, one maybe four years old and the other six-ish. The oldest is cordial and aloof; the youngest peppers me with questions.

"Do you own pets? Do you have children? Do you like them? Are any of them boys? Do you like berries? Do you want me to show you where they can be picked?"

The father finally interrupts and encourages his sons to continue walking. Long after they have disappeared around a bend I can hear the youngest boy shout to his father, "Daddy, I made a friend."

By the time I've returned to camp an imposing line of dark clouds is advancing and rain is falling. Not liking the vision of hunkering down under a steady downpour, I pull up the pegs, collapse the poles, cram the tent into its nylon bag, and text Cheryl to let her know I'm on my way home. As I head for the highway, the wind begins to blow rain sideways.

To the north a film of the deepest grey hangs like an enormous shower curtain drawn from horizon to horizon. I penetrate the curtain and the sky disappears. Wind bends the trees, clouds slope heavy and low and black over the landscape. The rain is fierce and unrelenting. The road becomes a thin, wet, shimmering ribbon. Lightning shears the darkness. The car shudders as thunder follows, and moments later I feel a fierce tug as the car is buffeted by a powerful blast of wind.

I grip the wheel, berating myself. I took the trip to clear my head, and I'm not sure that it's that much clearer as a result, and now it looks like I'll be vaporized by lightning or sucked up in a funnel cloud.

I should have let that boy show me where they picked the berries.

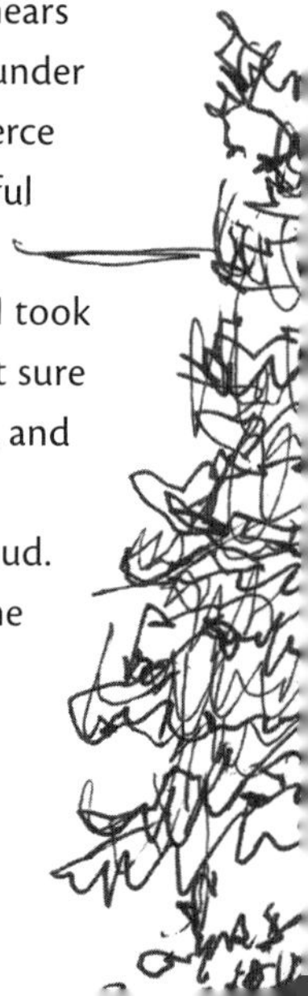

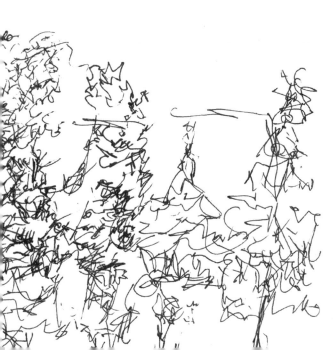

The storm breaks somewhere near Brooks and the rest of the drive is uneventful. But as I approach my neighbourhood, my wife calls to tell me that Liv is in trouble. His car is stalled in the middle of a road, and he has phoned her from some stranger's cell in a state of crisis. Cheryl remained on the line with him to keep him calm, but had to hang up to let him talk to whoever pulled over to help.

She gives me his location and as I drive up a road not far from his condominium, I spot his old white sedan blocking two lanes, and a middle-aged woman leaning through the driver's side window, talking to him. A child, who I assume to be her daughter, hangs back on the curb, looking nervous. I pull off the road, park, and walk over. When I tell the woman that I am Liv's brother, she looks relieved.

"Great," she says, and her voice drops. "I was worried. I didn't think I could leave him here, as he is, on his own, but I've got to get my daughter to her friend's place."

I shake her hand, thank her for her help, and then approach the car. Liv is seated, still gripping the steering wheel, face pale, sweating, in the midst of a serious panic attack. I lean in.

"Hi," I say. "I hear there's been some trouble. How are you doing?"

"Thank heavens you're here," he says.

"So, what's going on?"

"The car stopped in the middle of the road."

"Suddenly?"

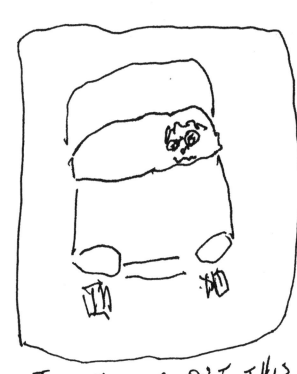

I TOOK CAR OUT THIS SUNDAY

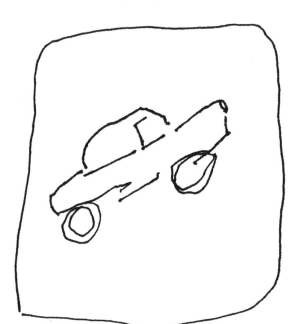

I KNEW IT WAS A MISTAKE SINCE MY CAR STALL IN TRAFFIC.

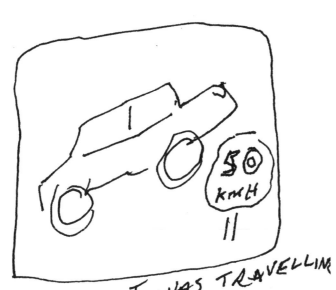

I KNEW I WAS TRAVELLING
FASTER THAN THE
SPEED LIMIT BUT
IF I SLOWED DOWN
IT WOULD STALL
THE HILL.

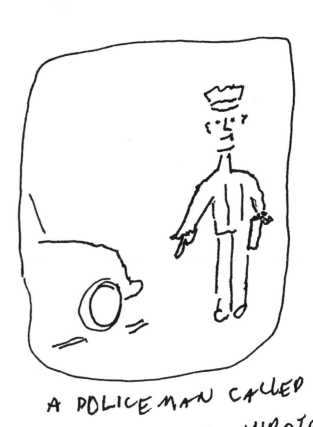

A POLICEMAN CALLED
ME OVER AND WROTE
A TICKET

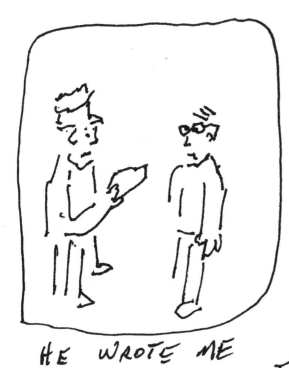

HE WROTE ME
A TICKET SAYING I
WAS GOING 68 KILOMETRES
IN A 50 CONSTRUCTION
ZONE

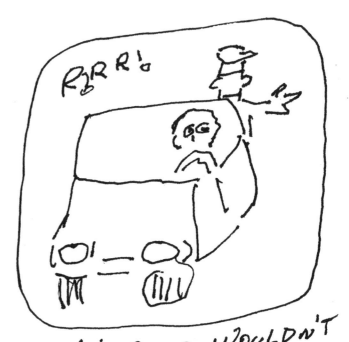

MY CAR WOULDN'T
START. I WAS
AFRAID I WOULD
GET ANOTHER
TICKET.

"Yes, suddenly."

"Did it stutter, or cut out, or wheeze?"

"It just stopped," he replies, beginning to get wound up, assuming that I'm questioning his judgment.

"Have you tried starting it again?"

"It won't start," he says, his voice rising, "I tried it—"

"Let's try it again," I say, wanting to keep the conversation calm, "and we'll listen together to find out if the motor turns over, or if the battery's dead." He places his key in the ignition. The motor catches and turns over.

"It wouldn't do that before," he says defensively.

"That's okay," I reassure him. "Whatever happened before, it's working now, that's the major thing. Drive it to your condominium and park it. If it looks like it's cutting out again, just pull over to the side of the road. I'll be right behind you."

He slips the car into gear. I climb into my car, turn it around, and follow him to the condominium parking lot. Liv stays in the car until I walk up and open the door.

"Can I borrow your cell phone? Mine died and I have to call the AMA," he says. "I called roadside assistance on that lady's phone and they'll be looking for me."

I tell him that we can go inside and call from his landline. He's just come back from an out-of-town retreat with a support group, so we unload his suitcases and sleeping bag and carry them up with us. Once he has cancelled the AMA roadside assistance, I offer him a glass of water, which he consumes thirstily. By the time I leave, everything is calm once again.

"Tell Cheryl I'm grateful she took my phone call," he says as I step into the hallway, "and thanks for helping me in my hour of need."

"I'll tell her," I assure him, and as I descend the stairs wonder if anyone else in the world says "hour of need."

On a chilly, clear October morning I drive to Olivier's place. Nic, Liv, and I are to gather at Liv's condominium for our six-month meeting with Dr. Baxter. Liv is in the living room, seated on the edge of the couch, looking anxious. He didn't sleep well, he says.

"Why?" I ask.

"I was worried that I wouldn't wake in time."

"What time did you get up?"

"Five."

"The appointment is at ten-thirty," I point out, and gesture behind him. "It's marked on your wall calendar."

"I became convinced that the appointment was at nine."

"That still doesn't explain why you felt you had to get up at five."

He shrugs. "I just did."

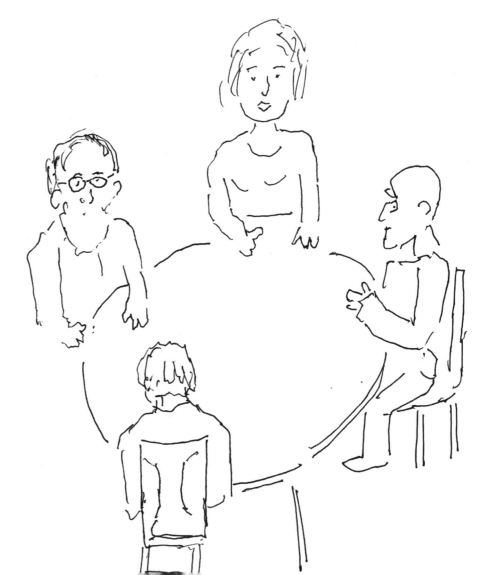

At that point, Nic arrives. The plan was for us to sit around the dining table and have tea, but the dining table is a catastrophe of old art supplies, used diabetes test strips, discarded coupons, and dirty dishes. Nic and I quickly collect and discard junk, pile assorted papers, and dust the chairs. I scrub some cups and saucers. The floor is littered with gravel and dirty clothes. While Olivier gathers them up, Nic vacuums up the gravel, and I tear off a strip of paper towel and wipe the table and kitchen counters. By the time Dr. Baxter arrives, there's at least a place for us to sit and rest our elbows.

She enters and, unconcerned by our flushed faces, greets us warmly, removes her coat, and drapes it over a chair. Olivier sits, clearly expecting some preliminary chitchat, but Dr. Baxter is eager to receive her promised tour. She claps her hands together and asks Olivier to show her around! He laughs nervously, rises from his chair and conducts her first on a circuit of the living room, the most organized of the living spaces. She nods in approval as she surveys the tidy coffee table surface, and the recently vacuumed carpet.

Next, he shows her Mom's old bedroom. This contains her mattress-less bed and her bureau, still stacked with tax documents, old letters, and knick-knacks. Dr. Baxter jots down a few notes and the tour rolls on. The spare room is crammed with drawings, felt pens, old paintings, old art supplies, a discarded computer, boxes of obsolete floppy disks, drawings, sculptures, and sketch pads.

He apologizes for the clutter, and then continues apologizing liberally throughout. First for the general disarray, and then several times as a precautionary measure prior to taking her into his disastrous bedroom. It is in a state of extreme disorder, almost unnavigable for the mountains of dirty laundry, teetering piles of books. What floor can be seen is littered with pens, cards, yellowing photos, dishes and cups, and unmatched running shoes. He halts a moment, not knowing what to say, but she urges him to carry on and take her through the kitchen. He apologizes once more as she opens the fridge – nearly empty but for a carton of milk, an unidentifiable vegetable, and a jar of what proves to be discoloured pickled beets.

The mysterious vegetable and jar of beets are immediately relegated to the garbage.

The cupboards are inhabited by a lonely can of beans, a half box of cereal, and an ancient bag of wheat germ.

"Why don't we sit down," Dr. Baxter suggests, "and have tea."

We assemble around the dining room table and fill our cups. As Dr. Baxter pours milk in her tea and stirs, she gently observes that grocery shopping seems to have slipped off the radar. Liv glumly agrees. She sips her tea and asks how he would assess his living conditions.

He purses his lips tightly and says, "I guess I'm not doing so well."

"Not so fast," she says. "Be a bit more specific. Where are you doing well, and where are you not?"

The conversation that follows is good and candid. Liv admits he's having trouble adjusting to life on his own. Dr. Baxter asks again if he would like a roommate. He thinks a moment then says that from what he has seen among his peers, roommates can be as much trouble as living alone. Dr. Baxter laughs and agrees with him.

"So, you want to continue working at it?" she asks.

Olivier pauses before he answers. "Yes."

I bring up Liv's recurring upset stomach, and the convulsions that sometimes hit him when he stands. She replies that Liv's medication can cause a variety of complications, but these symptoms, especially the convulsions, are odd. She'll order some tests.

She asks Nic and me if we helped clean the apartment before she arrived and when we confess that we did, she tells Olivier she'll arrange for Independent Living Skills to help him with housekeeping and groceries. When she rises to leave, Liv rises as well and thanks her. He tells her he doesn't believe he has ever had any other doctor pay a house call.

"I'm old-fashioned that way," she replies, grinning, as she slips on her jacket and leaves.

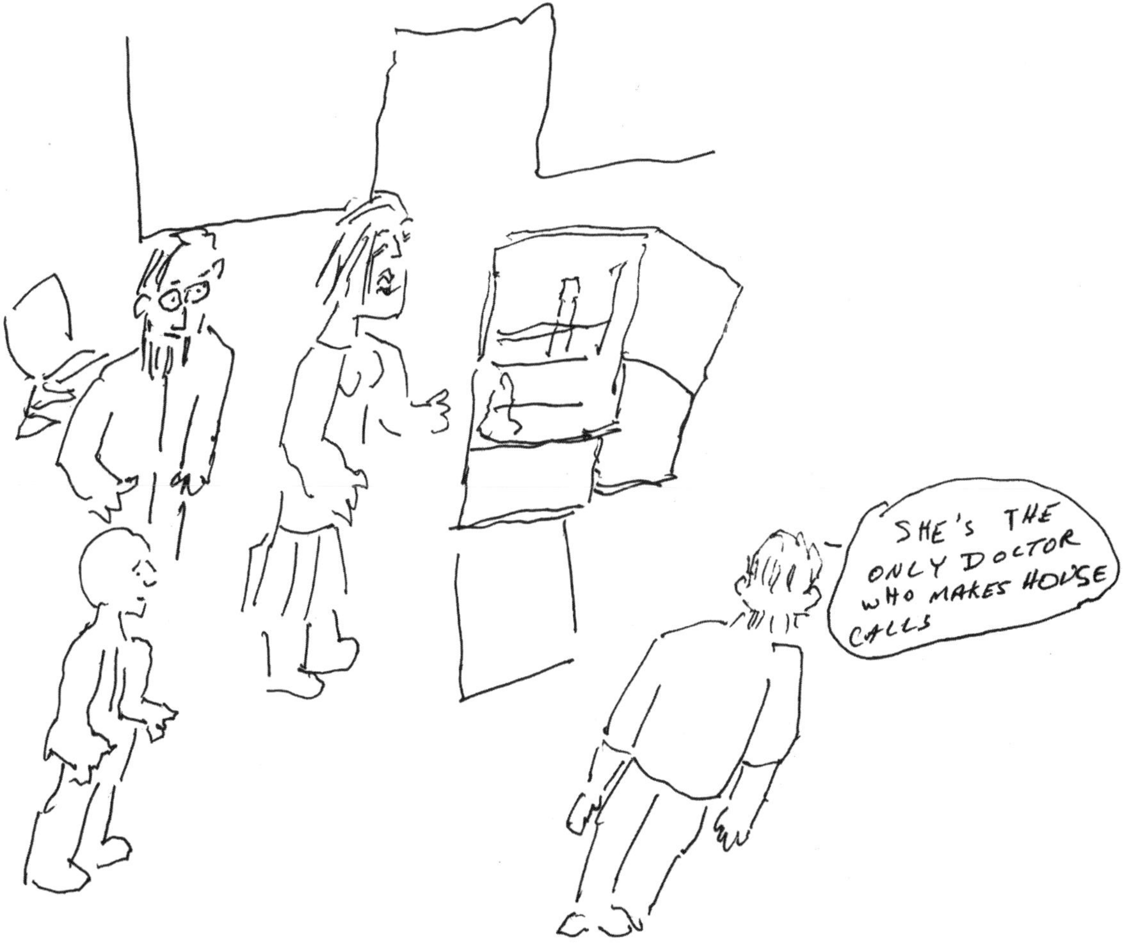
SHE'S THE ONLY DOCTOR WHO MAKES HOUSE CALLS

Before leaving the condo I do a little final tidying and discover a tiny note from my mother, tucked into a corner of the mantle in the living room, behind a brass clock. It's written on a torn scrap of paper, beginning first scrawled in crayon, then shifting to pen.

Will I ever see my sons to hear and see again? Or am I now out of their picture? They got purse (leather handbag and some money) all that is needed to even make a phone call! Whom did I kill, or threaten that I mustn't ever be allowed to phone them? Who decided to take away my citizenship, that it should become null and void? In case you want to get rid of me, just say so and prepare the Unitarian Church to have a memory for me. I love you all. If I hurt any of you, I am sorry, I did not mean to.

Your mother,
Catherine Martini

How long, I wonder, did she sit and wrestle with her delusions? How many more desperate, lonely notes did she draft and discard in the nooks and crannies of the apartment?

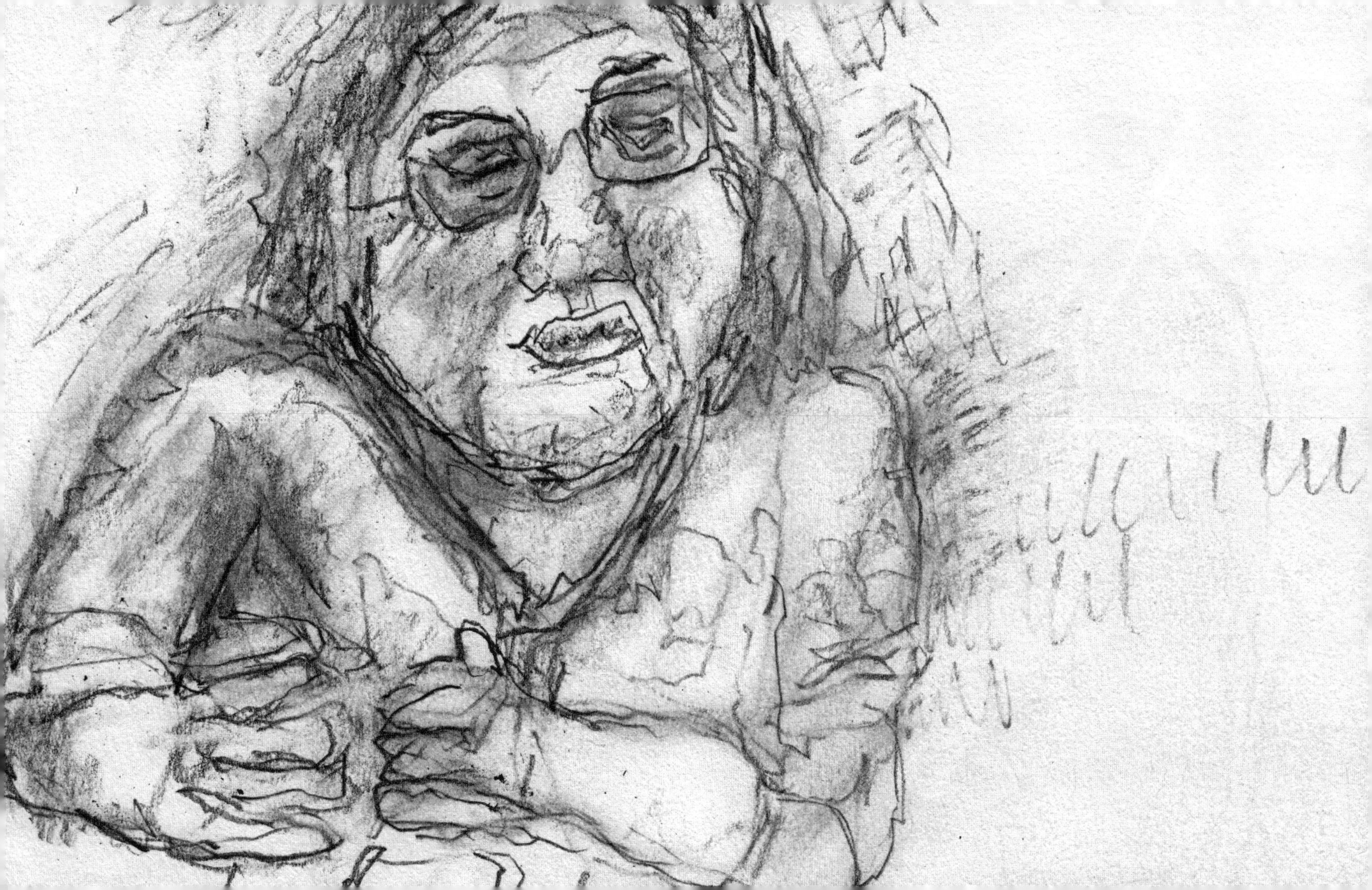

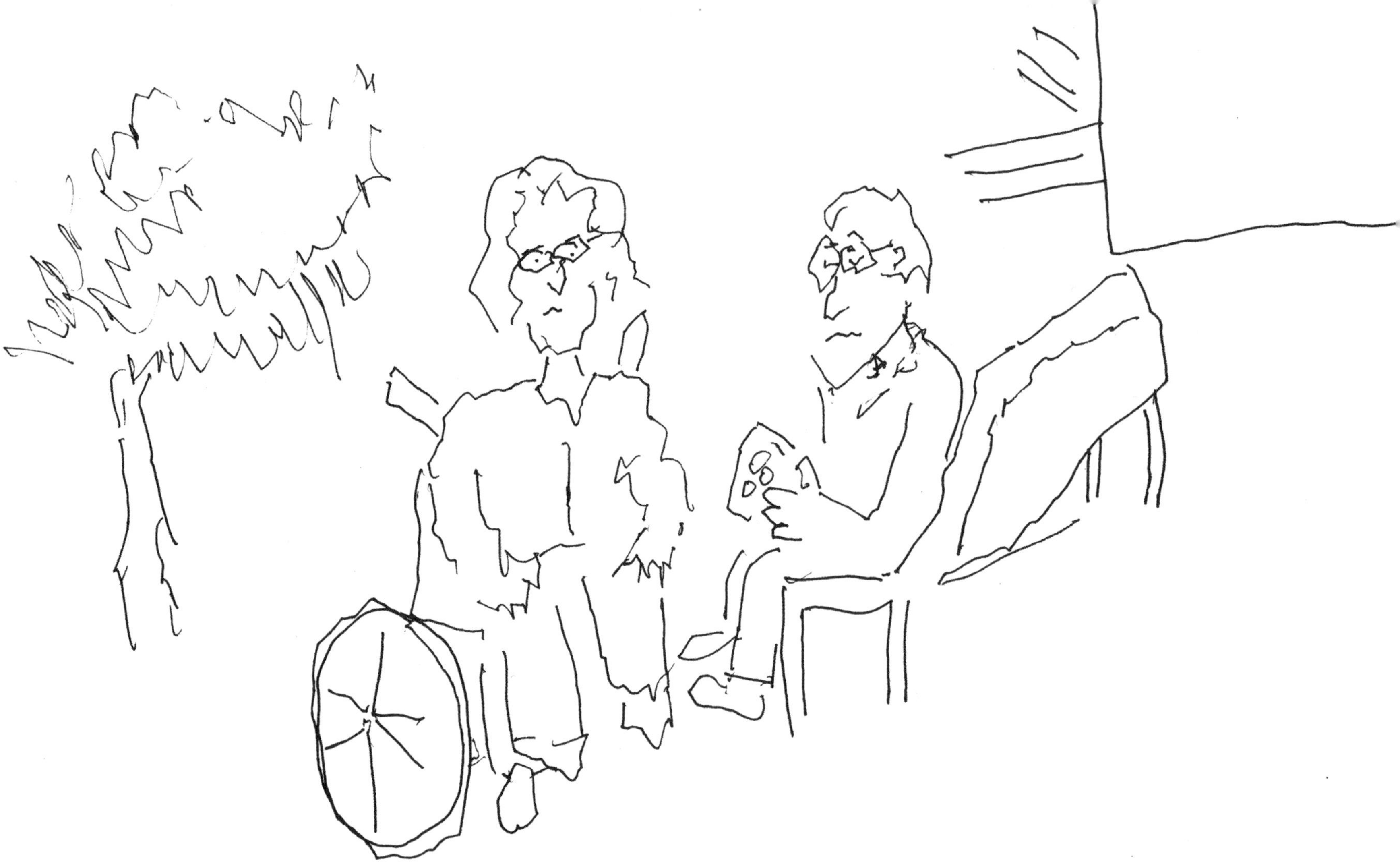

I sit in my living room and watch the sun rise, gilding the needles of the pines in the front yard gold. It's clear and cold outside, ice crystals shimmering in the air. As I slip my coat on in preparation to leave for the Bow Valley, Cher emerges from the kitchen and tosses me a mandarin orange. I thank her and tuck it in my coat pocket.

When I enter my mother's bedroom, she stares blankly at me and has trouble putting words together. When I suggest that we go downstairs for coffee, her face remains empty. I'm not sure she knows who I am.

Then abruptly she smiles and is transformed. It is as though her mind has slowly retraced its steps and come across a cache of forgotten, happy memories. I wheel her downstairs. We lounge in a patch of sunlight in the courtyard. I take the mandarin orange out of my pocket and peel it, and she methodically separates the pith from the fruit. I show her some photos on my phone. She observes them with interest, but doesn't comment. She asks if I will cut her nails, which have grown quite long. I leave her with some coffee to drink, return to her room, and fetch the nail clippers and a file. We spend the next half hour doing her nails. One of the residents, a woman seated in a wheelchair across the courtyard, watches intently the whole time, then comments that my mother is lucky. As usual, my mother can't hear and asks that I repeat what the woman said. I do, and my mother grins and says she knows she is lucky.

I wheel her to her room and put the nail clippers and file away. I tell my mother I will return on Sunday – I don't know if she'll remember. She probably won't. She smiles and wishes me a good night.

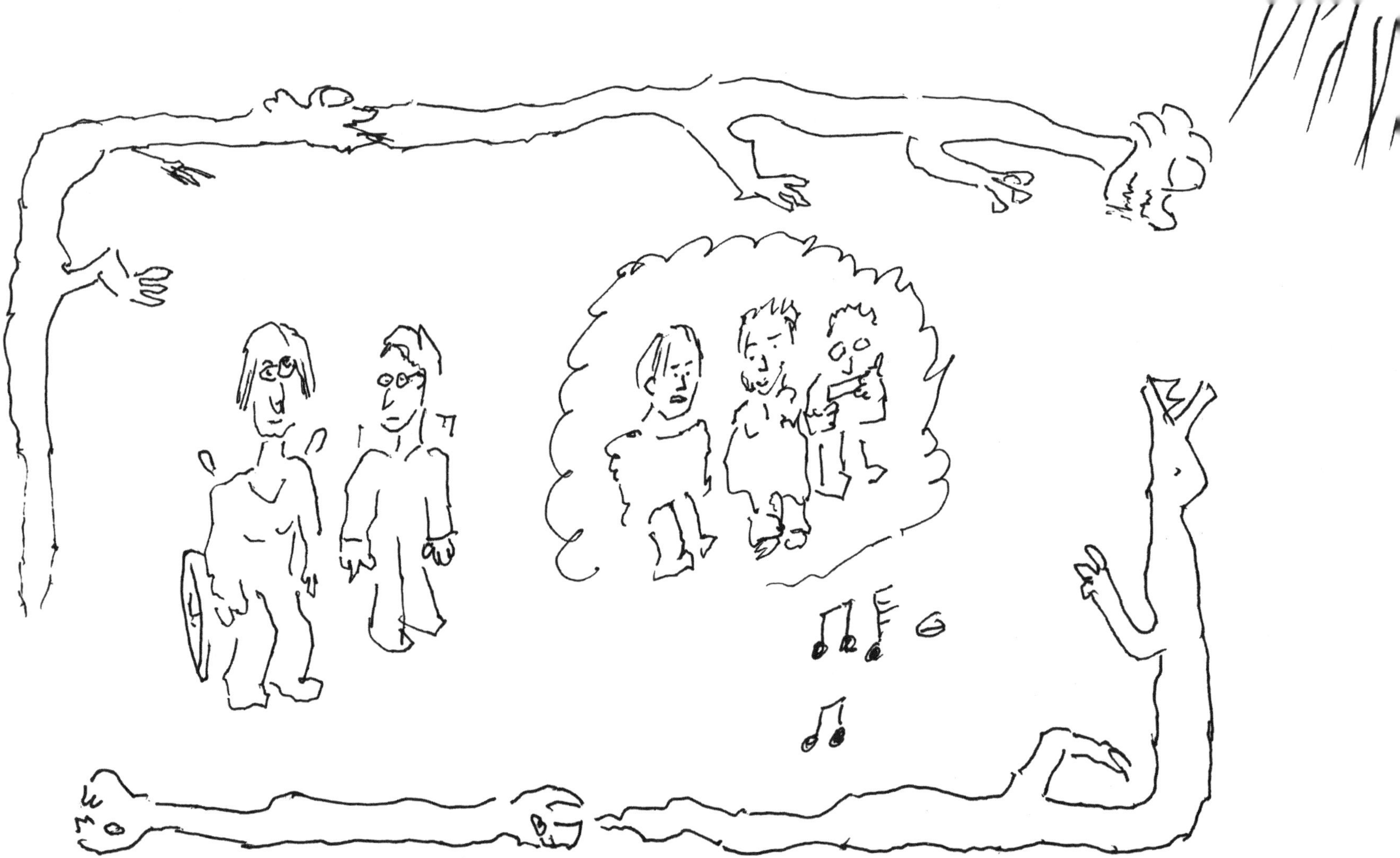

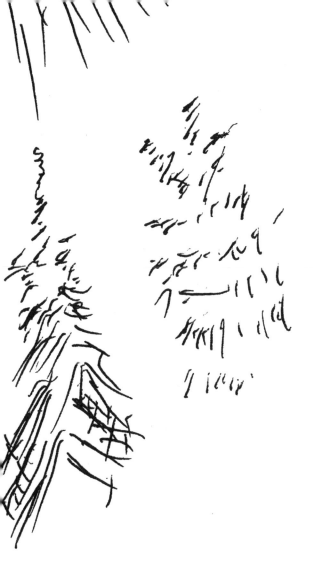

Tonight we attend the Bow Valley Christmas Dinner, my mother, my brothers, and I. It seems a little premature, falling as it does on December 8, but I suppose it's scheduled that way to guarantee that sufficient staff are on hand.

Nic, Liv, and I mount the stairs to the second floor and find Mom in her room. She has selected, or had selected on her behalf, a nice burgundy-coloured blouse for the occasion. We wheel her into the elevator and then out to the courtyard, which is festooned with cutout snowflakes strung from multicoloured streamers. Blue and white Christmas lights dangle and glitter from the branches above us. An adult-sized snowman, crafted of Styrofoam cups, grins a greeting. Round dinner tables draped with white linen stand among the trees of the courtyard.

We find a handwritten place card — *Catherine Martini and family* — at a table beneath the broad leaves of an enormous rubber plant, and take our seats beside two brothers whose mother and father were both residents at the Bow Valley at one time. Their parents have since died, but the brothers tell us they feel like this place has become a kind of second home for them. They return every Christmas to help out and participate in the banquet. An elderly lady in an electronic wheelchair arrives with a soft hum of the motor and parks herself at the table alongside her husband and grown daughter.

217

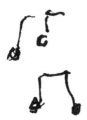

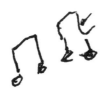

There's some initial confusion about how best to position my mother's wheelchair at the table. Mom doesn't respond well to last-minute adjustments so at first she's a bit on edge, but once the bread bowl is passed around she begins to relax. Staff come around serving punch thick with chopped fruit. It's sweet, just to my mother's taste. She swiftly downs her first cup, devours the fruit, and requests more.

There's the usual trouble with her deafness. She can't really hear anyone apart from the person beside her and feels left out if she can't converse with all of us, so we rotate who sits next to her throughout the dinner, which assures she has an opportunity to talk with each of us one-on-one at some point.

The meal arrives still steaming: turkey, mashed potatoes, gravy, dressing, green beans, and a bun — simple but nicely cooked. We offer Christmas toasts then everyone eats and chats. Once our main course is cleared away, we're served fruitcake and tea. Following the dinner, a band sets up and plays selections from the fifties and sixties. I am pleasantly surprised to see how much the music delights my mother. She's never been particularly fond of the Beatles or Roy Orbison — I don't believe she even knows who Roy Orbison was — but tonight she claps her hands and slaps the tabletop in time with the music as though she was their biggest fan. I exchange grins with my brothers, who are similarly caught off guard. Her unexpected enthusiasm and genuine pleasure constitute a bit of a Bow Valley Christmas miracle, and in that instant I feel fortunate. Fortunate to have the brothers I have, the mother I have, and to share this moment with them.

A woman behind us nearly upsets her table when she uses the tablecloth to wipe her mouth. An elderly couple at the table to our left rise, embrace and slow dance. Nic, Liv and I hang on till the party has begun to thin out, then return Mom to her room. She is exhausted but happy. We hug and wish her a merry Christmas.

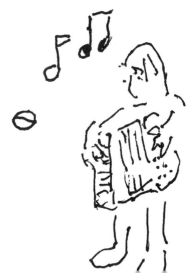

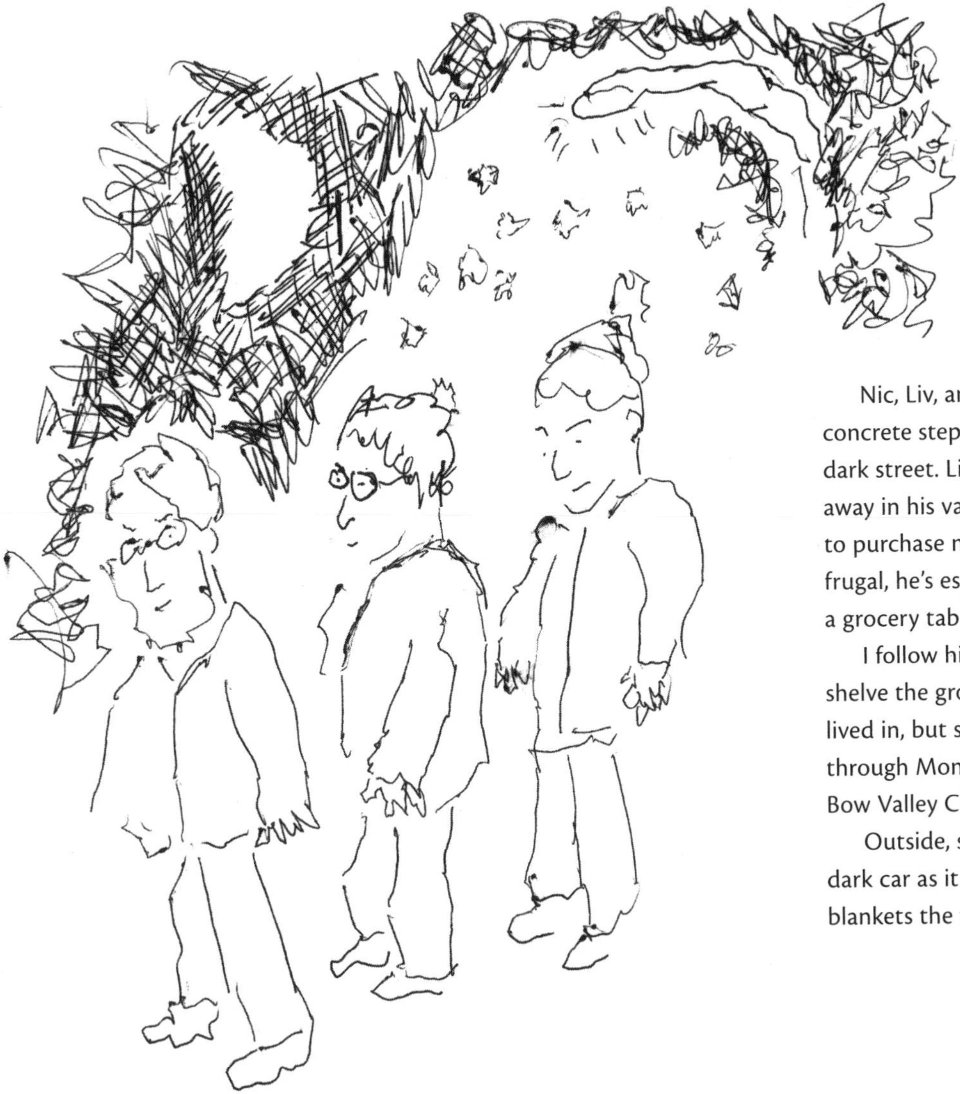

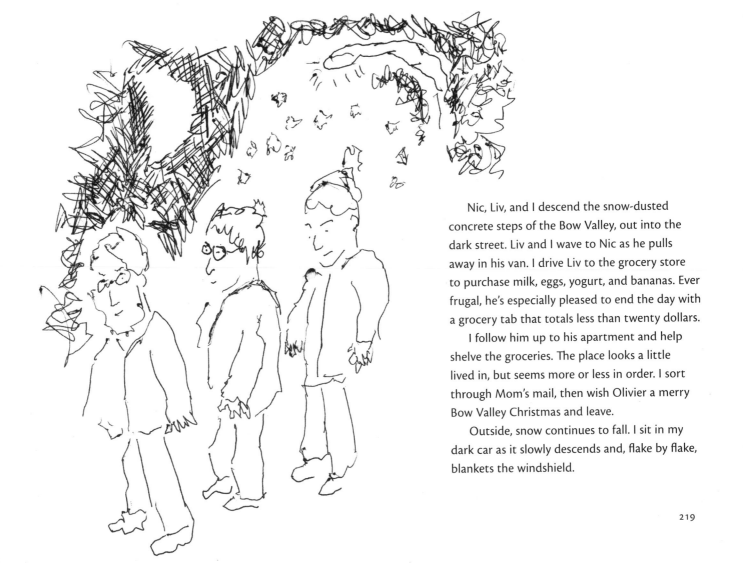

Nic, Liv, and I descend the snow-dusted concrete steps of the Bow Valley, out into the dark street. Liv and I wave to Nic as he pulls away in his van. I drive Liv to the grocery store to purchase milk, eggs, yogurt, and bananas. Ever frugal, he's especially pleased to end the day with a grocery tab that totals less than twenty dollars.

I follow him up to his apartment and help shelve the groceries. The place looks a little lived in, but seems more or less in order. I sort through Mom's mail, then wish Olivier a merry Bow Valley Christmas and leave.

Outside, snow continues to fall. I sit in my dark car as it slowly descends and, flake by flake, blankets the windshield.

In my dream Olivier is about to cross the ocean in a canoe and I will, apparently, accompany him. We'll travel thousands of miles without the benefit of either motor or sail. I'm daunted by the proposition, although not as daunted as I would be in reality. There's trouble of some kind acquiring the canoe, but in the way of dreams, suddenly we are in it, paddling. Navigating the swells of the open ocean proves challenging, although curiously this is the easiest portion of the dream.

We eventually arrive at a remote, tropical island community, and transfer to a longer boat where we find my mother and Nic. My mother sits in the stern, serene, oblivious to the efforts of others or the dangers of the water, while the rest of us paddle. After another much shorter journey we tie up at a harbour that hosts an enormous fresh fruit market. As we make our way through the crowded stalls, Nic complains that it's mostly grapefruit being sold and then, again in the way of dreams, we're separated.

And suddenly it's dark and I am rowing back alone. I have to retrace the route across the ocean and can't remember my way.

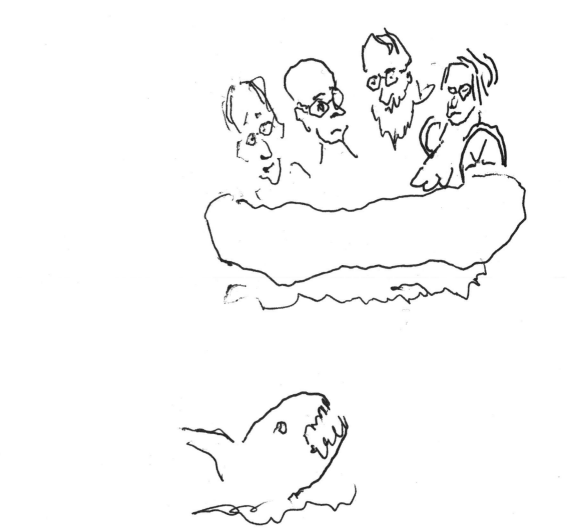

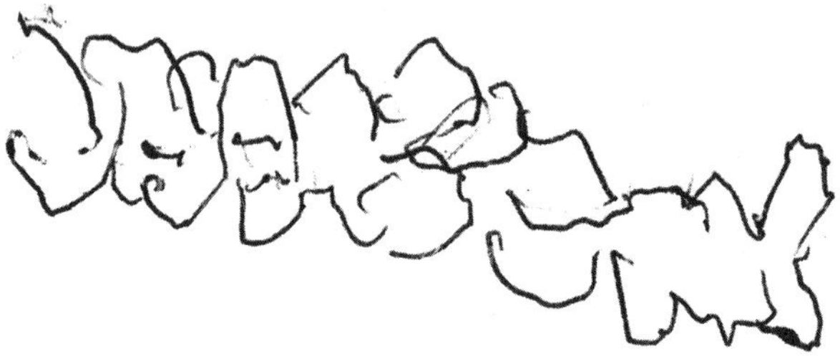

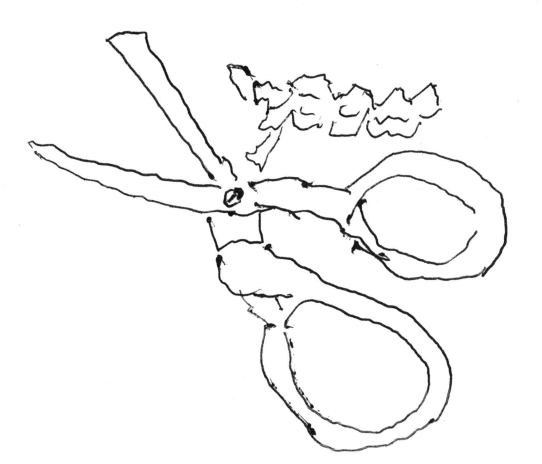

After my brother Olivier was first diagnosed with schizophrenia, he experienced some very difficult years. The illness, the side effects of the medication, the alienation he felt, and the depression were crushing. He stayed at home with my mother, who supported him, encouraged him to take his meds, made him get up each morning, got on his nerves several times a day, but genuinely helped. Until one day, she couldn't.

When we realized that the system we had was unravelling I thought at first it would be possible to mend it, to find a clean, tidy remedy for each of the separate problems. I was wrong. You can fly at the problems that face you and miss every one.

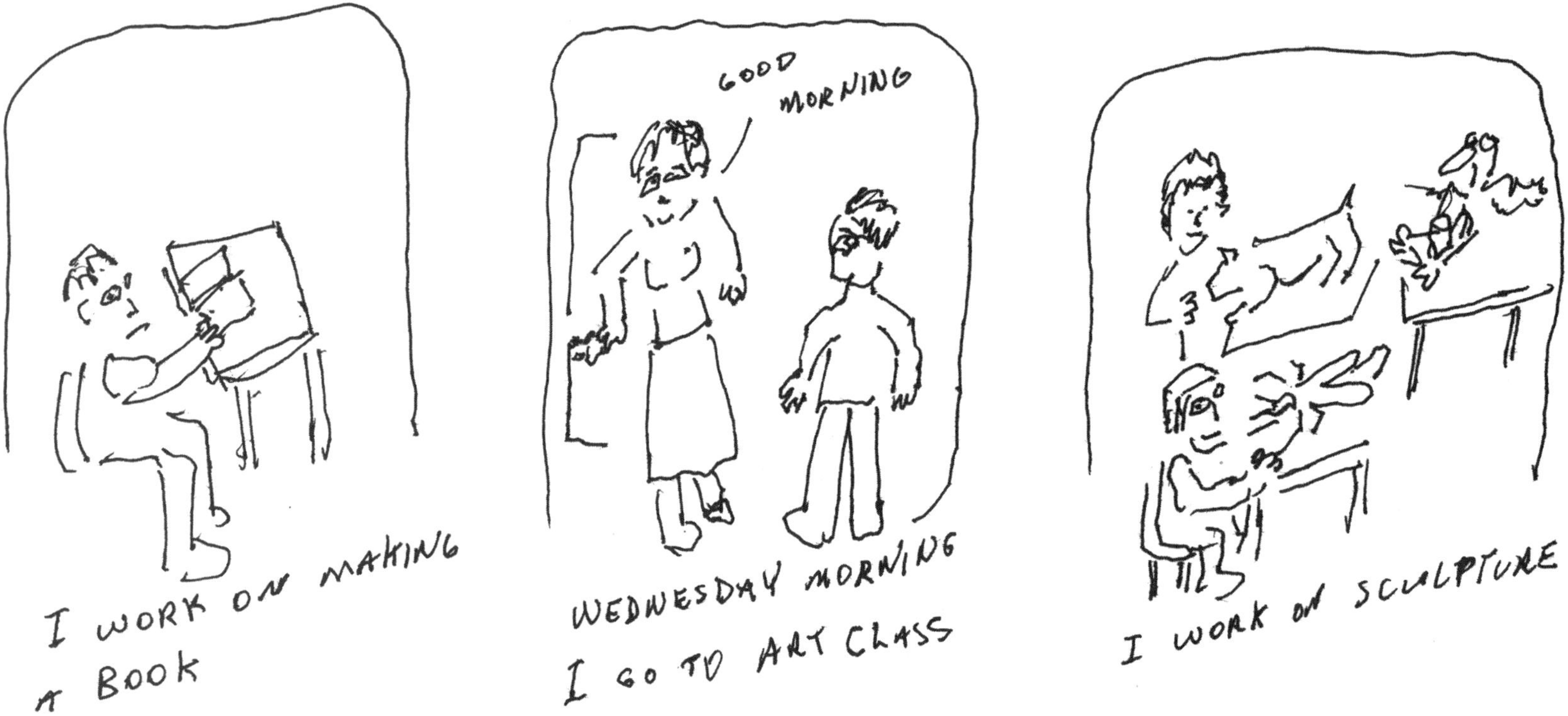
I WORK ON MAKING A BOOK
GOOD MORNING
WEDNESDAY MORNING
I GO TO ART CLASS
I WORK ON SCULPTURE

At first, to the degree that it was possible, I tried to keep my family, my wife and children, at a distance from the messiness that emerged, as I judged it too chaotic, and potentially too damaging. Luckily for me, they resisted my efforts. They were patient, gave me space when I required it, stepped in when it was necessary, and in general helped me to maintain my sanity.

Olivier has had to do the hardest work, and there have been times when I think this transition has been the fight of his life, but I believe he has pulled through. Finding a way to adapt and reorganize has been an enormous struggle, but he's a resourceful, stubborn individual and he has managed to develop a new lifestyle that works for him. He sold his car because he felt anxious looking after it and panicky driving it. He takes CTrains and buses now and is happier for it. He maintains the apartment — it's never going to appear on the cover of *Home and Design Magazine* but it doesn't need to. He doesn't buy much, and keeps things simple, which given his propensity for clutter is probably wise. Independent Living Skills has stepped in, helping with housekeeping and ensuring he takes his meds and meals on schedule. He exercises at the Y, maintains his art practice, participates in a variety of groups, and socializes with his peers. Most days, nearly every day, he visits our mother. At one time he felt guilty about her circumstances, but I think he's accepted that the situation at the apartment was untenable.

His illness requires watching, and flares up unexpectedly, but to a good degree, he attends to it. We talk most days. If things fail, Nic and I, his extended family, his health care team, and his friends in the community are there.

As for my mother, I wish so many things. I wish my grandmother, who I never met, hadn't died when my mother was still a child. I wish that my mother's one-armed father had been less stern, more compassionate, had been able to genuinely care for a daughter who was grieving the loss of a parent. I wish that my mother hadn't been conscripted to fight in a war when she was still a teenager, hadn't lost all her extended family to bombing. I wish there hadn't been a need for her to be so independent so young.

I wish we could have negotiated her transition to nursing care more easily. I wish she
could let go of her fierce desire for independence and accept help. More than anything else
I wish she could be happier. I still feel the urge
to whisper in her ear, "Just be different, and
your experience with dementia could be better.
You could be the happy, confused older
person that the nursing staff love to coddle.
You could be the one who forgets things, but
for whom the staff are eager to fetch coffee
and a butter tart." But that's not going to
happen. My mother is never going to become
the sweet, forgetful, forgiving resident. She is
who she is — and each day she is less of that.

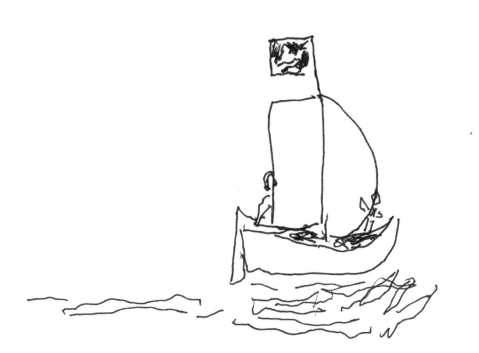

Conclusion

You think you are in control of your life. You believe you have a notion of how the future is unfolding. And then one day everything comes apart — all your plans so much vapour.

There are a million earnest, desperately unprepared, underqualified families providing care for ill or aging relatives the best way they know how, improvising solutions for medical troubles they have never been trained to recognize or treat — an enormous number of them ill or aging themselves. They are hanging on as best they can, but they need help.

Hospitals can barely accommodate the present numbers, let along hope to accommodate the numbers of aged looming on the horizon. And as all these people that the government relies upon to perform caregiving in their homes falter, as surely they will, how will the health care system cope? So far the government's answer appears to be a million phone lines primed to place you on hold, or transfer you to their non-existent answering services. The Alzheimer's Society of Canada says that 564,000 Canadians currently live with dementia and in fifteen years that will increase to 937,000; many of those almost one million individuals are presently caregivers themselves. We are in this, we are all the way in, and believe me, we are in this together.

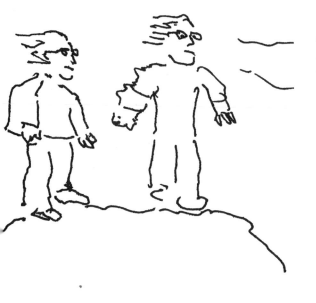

In 2012 following the release of our book *Bitter Medicine: A Graphic Memoir of Mental Illness*, Olivier and I were invited to meet with the University of Calgary's first-year nursing class to discuss education relating to mental health issues. *Bitter Medicine* deals with my family's experience with schizophrenia and the challenges we faced living on the edges of the mental health care system.

The students told us they had read our book, were moved by it, and found it enormously helpful — they hadn't understood what mental illness was like from the perspective of families dealing with it, and were beginning to see the ways that the medical system falls short. The only way to improve the conditions of care, as far as they could see, was if people who have had experience, like Liv and me, speak up. Patients, and families of patients, will have to open up and share their stories, they said, because the public genuinely doesn't understand mental illness.

That's true. But who really wants to share these stories, in many cases their worst stories? What do you stand to gain? You are tarred forever in the public's perception. It's not a noble, uplifting experience living with mental illness or dementia. It's not the noble or uplifting stories that will change the way things operate either: it's the stories that are uncomfortable, disturbing, embarrassing, unsettling, the ones that people all over the country find themselves living secretly every single day.

There are many, many people who find themselves in situations like the ones I've described, who realize their circumstances are no longer sustainable but possess no back-up plan and no additional resources. The governments of this country, federal and provincial, have turned to family caregiving as the go-to solution for those struggling with mental illnesses. But what happens when that solution collapses? What happens when caregivers grow too old to provide care, or get ill and require care themselves? We're finding out now.

My family's story is still in progress. We're in the middle. And the middle is by definition a mess. It's unfinished. There's no tidiness or clarity to it. Loose threads dangle everywhere. And I worry about when exactly I should share our stories. At what state of readiness? Part of me wants to wait until I know how it will all turn out, until I know that we've done the right thing. Part of me is scared. What if I get it wrong? What if I tell it wrong? What if the exposure proves too great? And part of me says, screw it, tell it now.

Because I feel a tremendous sense of urgency. My family and I have spent a lifetime struggling with mental health issues of one form or another in a health care system that doesn't get it, doesn't work, that wants family caregivers to take up the slack, and when they can't, always, always leaves you feeling like it could have worked if only you and your family weren't such total screw-ups in the first place. I confess that I have spent a lifetime feeling ashamed. Ashamed of the embarrassing, awkward activities that necessarily accompany mental illness and dementia. The inappropriate interactions. Loud late-night arguments. Fistfights in public. Pacing in emergency waiting rooms, racing after family members fleeing from psychiatric wards. Ashamed that I couldn't do enough to save my younger brother from suicide. Crushed that my older brother has lived a life of diminished hopes. Embarrassed that I'm not wealthy enough to fix things, ashamed that I'm not Zen enough to be unashamed. And always, always waiting for the right time to speak.

But I am through waiting.

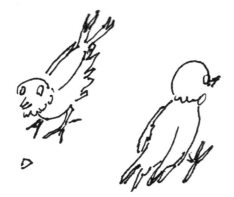

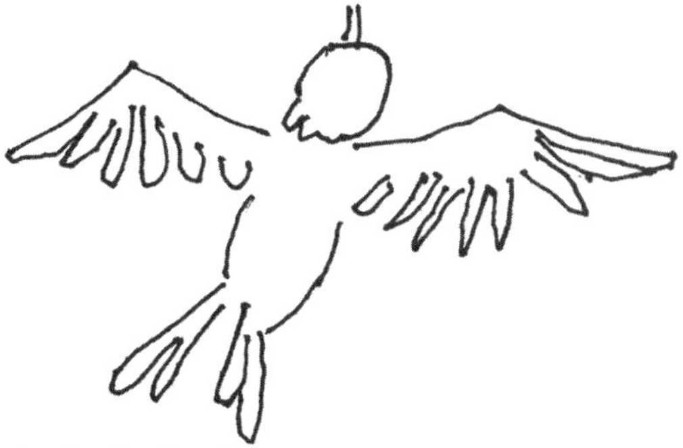

Epilogue

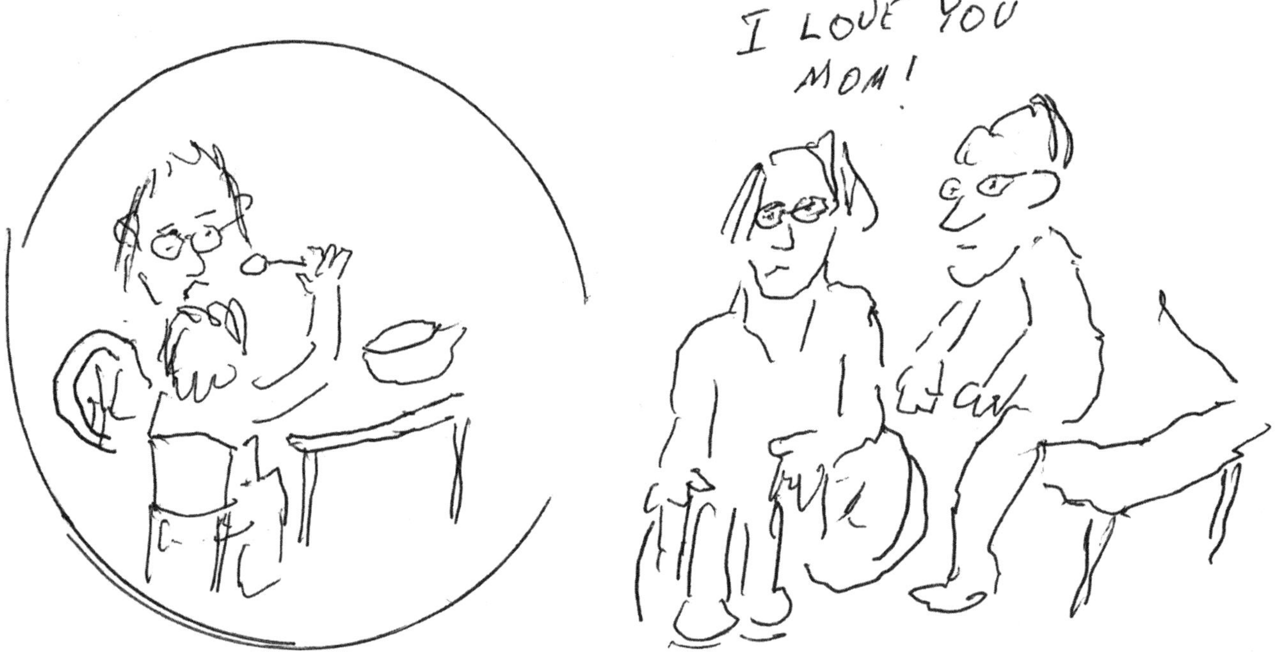
I LOVE YOU MOM!

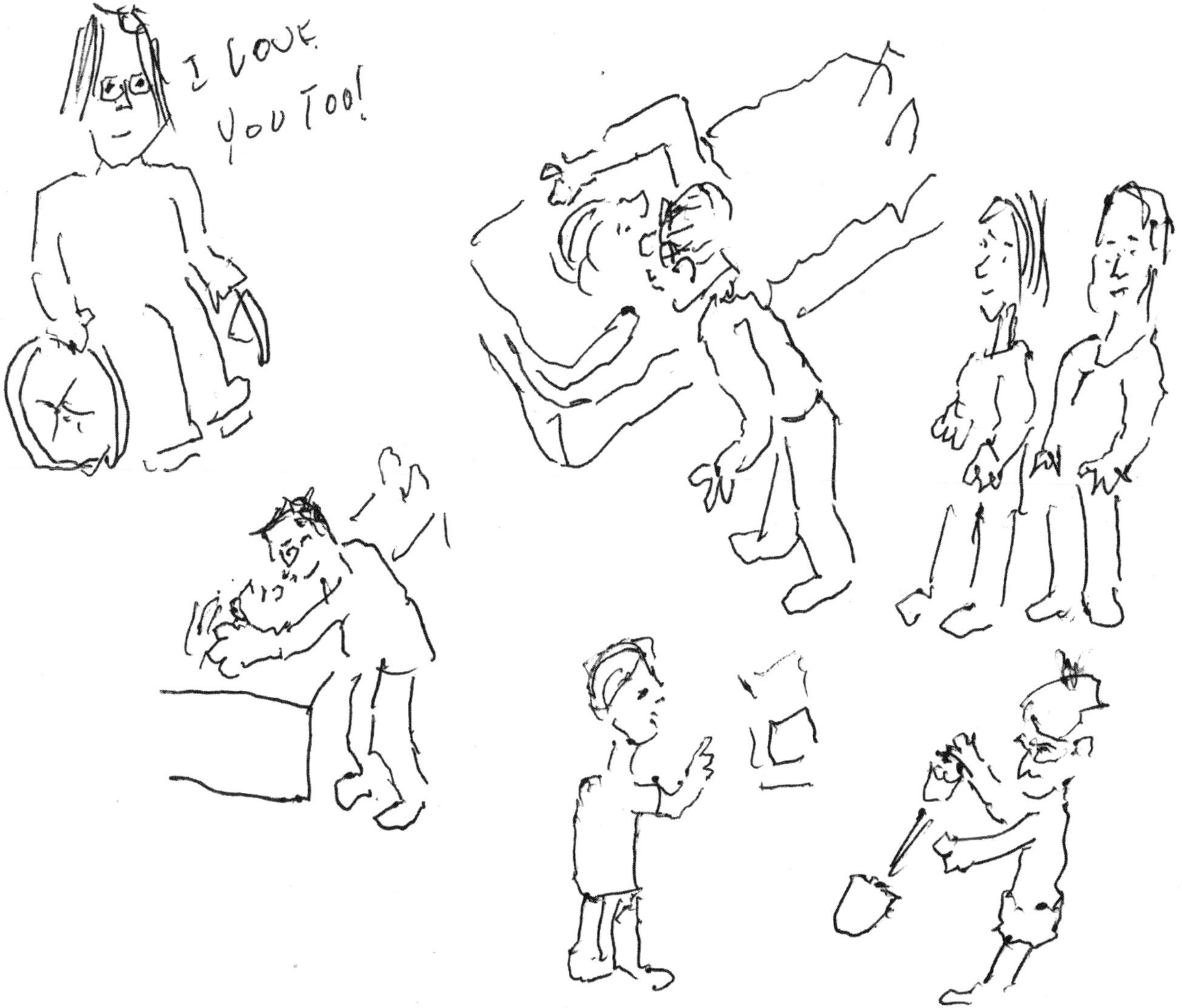
I LOVE YOU TOO!

I'm just leaving work when I receive a phone call from the Bow Valley. The voice on the other end informs me that my mother has contracted a fever. Can I come down?

She's alone in her room when I arrive, stretched flat upon her bed, eyes closed, one thin hand extended beyond the blanket, clutching the metal guardrail. Plastic tubes snake up her nose. Her mouth gapes, and her breathing emerges in painfully slow, regular gasps.

"Mom?" I say.

She doesn't stir, so I sit beside the bed and place my hand upon hers. It's warm and papery smooth. I watch her breathe, and wait for the resident doctor to complete his rounds.

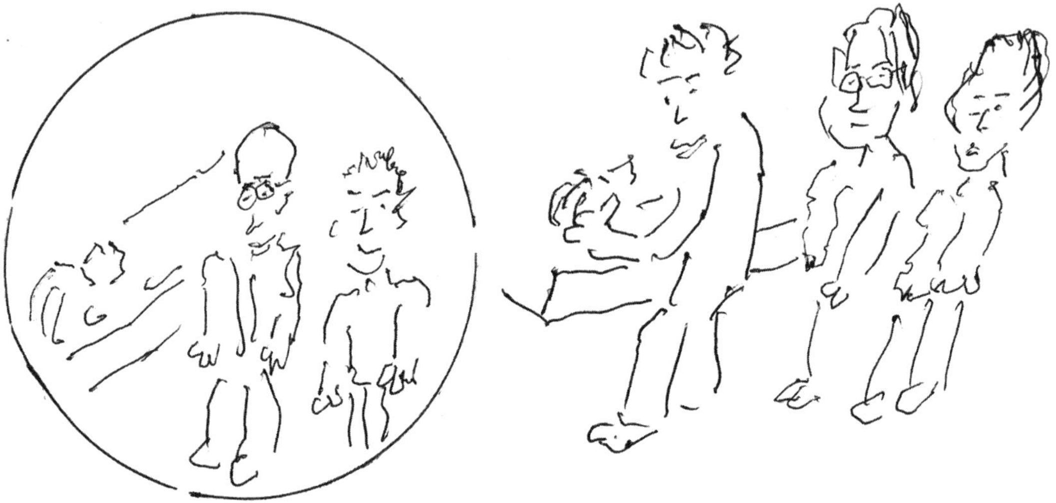

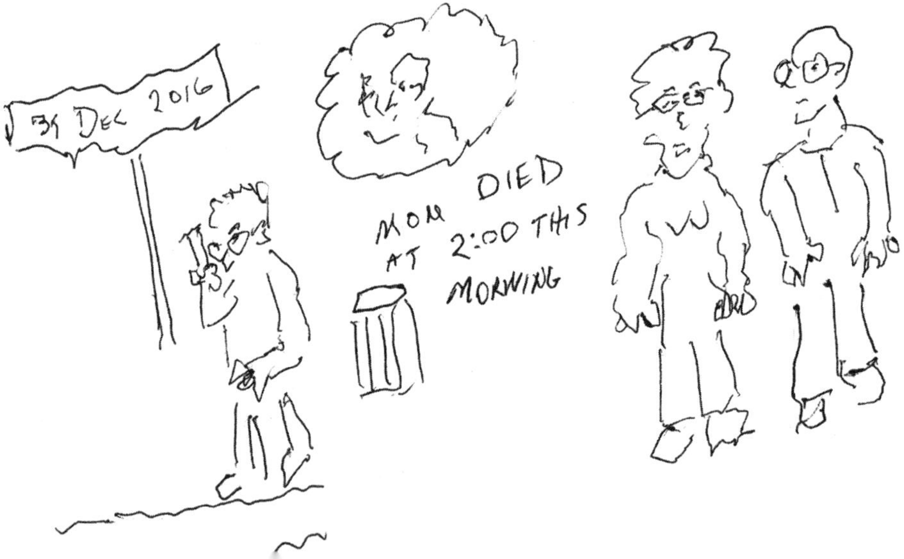
31 DEC 2016
MOM DIED AT 2:00 THIS MORNING

"Pneumonia," he tells me when he arrives. She took to her bed early last night, then wasn't able to rise for breakfast. The staff did what they could to make her comfortable, providing painkillers and oxygen.

He's seen this kind of thing happen many times, he tells me. "It can progress rapidly, and it's hard to say for sure how things will develop," he observes as he watches her. "It's possible that she will pull out of it, but she's ninety-one." He leaves that thought dangling.

I call my brothers and wife and inform them of the situation. Cheryl, Chandra, Miranda, and Liv join me later that evening. My daughters sing to their grandmother, and she briefly opens her eyes and smiles. Nic and his family arrive a little later.

At 2:45 a.m. she stops breathing.

And it's amazing to me that something can be both completely expected, and at the same time such a disorienting jolt. There are no last words; death permits no second chances. There's just the stillness of the room and the sad realization that she is gone.

I bid her goodbye. I lean over the bed to closely consider her face. The deep lines of anxiety, confusion and anger that developed with the onset of dementia seem to relax, and in that quiet, final moment it's possible to imagine my mother as she once was.

Catherine Martini 1925–2016

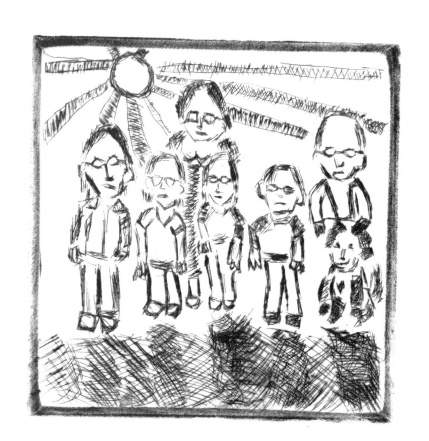

Published with the generous assistance of the
Canada Council for the Arts and the Alberta
Media Fund.

Canada Council   Conseil des Arts
for the Arts   du Canada

Alberta
Government

Freehand Books
515 – 815 1st Street SW
Calgary, Alberta
T2P 1N3
www.freehand-books.com

Book orders: LitDistCo
8300 Lawson Road
Milton, Ontario
L9T 0A4
T: 1-800-591-6250
F: 1-800-591-6251
E: orders@litdistco.ca
www.litdistco.ca

Edited by Barbara Scott
Book design by Natalie Olsen, Kisscut Design
Printed on FSC recycled paper and bound
in Canada by Friesens

Library and Archives Canada Cataloguing in Publication

Martini, Clem, 1956–, author
The unravelling : how our caregiving safety net came unstrung and
we were left grasping at threads, struggling to plait a new one /
Clem Martini and Olivier Martini.

Issued in print and electronic formats.
ISBN 978-1-988298-15-3 (softcover).
ISBN 978-1-988298-16-0 (epub).
ISBN 978-1-988298-17-7 (pdf)

1. Martini, Olivier — Mental health — Comic books, strips, etc.
2. Martini, Olivier — Family — Comic books, strips, etc.
3. Schizophrenics — Family relationships — Comic books, strips, etc.
4. Mental health services — Alberta — Comic books, strips, etc.
5. Schizophrenics — Canada — Biography — Comic books, strips, etc.
6. Biographical comics.
I. Martini, Olivier, illustrator
II. Title.

RC514.M378 2017   616.89'800922   C2017-903720-X   C2017-903721-8

Praise for
Bitter Medicine: A Graphic Memoir of Mental Illness

"[A] poignant, heart-wrenching and at times infuriating story about the Martini family's 30-year battles with schizophrenia and the mental health-care system."
— *Calgary Herald*

"The book's greatest strength is its profound ability to humanize a frequently misunderstood condition, and to highlight mental illness as the 'orphan child' of the health care community."
— *Quill and Quire*

"Much is lost because of mental illness. With books like *Bitter Medicine*, much is gained."
— *The Coast*

"This is a rare and powerful book. It gives the meaning of love without talking of love. It is both heartbreaking and truly victorious. It tells us clearly that mental illness is a dimension of 'normal' the way that shadow is a dimension of light. And we should walk with our shadows."
— **Dragan Todorovic, author of** *The Book of Revenge*

"[A] meaningful look into the difficulties and guilt that assuage everyday families who have to deal with a family member with schizophrenia. . . What resonates in this book is the frustration that the Martinis feel at the hands of our health care system and the bond that this family forges."
— *Broken Pencil*

"The inclusion of Olivier's drawings offers an illuminating presence often missing from mental health discussions. They make Olivier's story heartbreakingly real, lending credence to Clem's shattering facts about mental health. The format also makes light reading of heavy issues, and imparts a page-turning interest to deliver the importance of them."
— *Telegraph-Journal*

"There's hope in the art of Olivier, whose line drawings evoke the work of R.O. Blechman. Though much of the work — some old, some produced for the book — is bleak, he infuses a remarkable amount of humour and joy into his drawings."
— *National Post*